Welcome to

THE
EVERYTHING®

HEALTH GUIDES

When you're faced with a pressing health issue, your first instinct is to find out as much about it as you can. With so much conflicting information out there, where can you turn for professional, supportive advice?

Packed with the most recent, up-to-date data, THE EVERYTHING® HEALTH GUIDES help ensure that you get a good diagnosis, choose the best doctor, and find the right medical treatment. With this one comprehensive resource, you and your family members have all the information you could possibly need—at your fingertips.

THE EVERYTHING® HEALTH GUIDES are an extension of the best-selling Everything® series in the health category, which also includes *The Everything® Diabetes Book* and *The Everything® Menopause Book*. Accessible and easy to read, THE EVERYTHING® HEALTH GUIDES provide specific details and clear examples that relate to your given medical situation. If you're looking for one-stop, all-inclusive guides that allow you to understand and become more in tune with your body, this groundbreaking series is the perfect tool for you.

Visit the entire Everything® series at *www.everything.com*

THE EVERYTHING

HEALTH GUIDE TO
Adult Bipolar Disorder

Dear Reader,

Bipolar disorder affects the lives of millions of people. Whether you are bipolar yourself, know someone who is, or are simply are curious to know more about it, I hope you will find this book a helpful and informative resource.

In many ways, writing this book was like a juggling act. Professionals will verify the extreme importance of staying on medication and the tragic consequences that can occur when patients do not. This can make the disorder seem like a very grave affliction. But at the same time, there is strong reason for hope and optimism found in the bipolar people who live normal and fulfilling lives. In fact, there are many bipolar people who achieve fame and fortune and who make a real contribution to society.

If the message of this book had to be summarized in a single phrase, it would be: "Stay on medication." But hopefully, this guide will inform bipolar people and their loved ones about a wide range of issues regarding the disorder and impact their lives in a positive way.

Jon P. Bloch, Ph.D.

THE

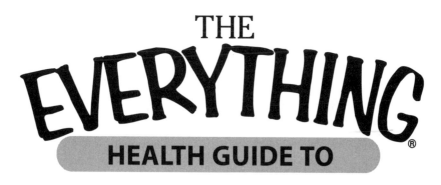

EVERYTHING

HEALTH GUIDE TO

ADULT BIPOLAR DISORDER

Reassuring advice to help you cope

Jon P. Bloch, Ph.D.

with Technical Review by Jeffrey A. Naser, M.D.

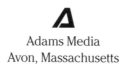

Adams Media
Avon, Massachusetts

Dedication

To all the people I have known who live outside the box.

• • •

Publishing Director: Gary M. Krebs
Associate Managing Editor: Laura M. Daly
Associate Copy Chief: Brett Palana-Shanahan
Acquisitions Editor: Kate Burgo
Development Editor: Katie McDonough
Associate Production Editor: Casey Ebert
Technical Reviewer: Jeffrey A. Naser, M.D.

Director of Manufacturing: Susan Beale
Associate Director of Production: Michelle Roy Kelly
Cover Design: Paul Beatrice, Erick DaCosta, Matt LeBlanc
Layout and Graphics: Colleen Cunningham, Holly Curtis, Sorae Lee

An Everything® Series Book.
Everything® and everything.com® are registered trademarks of F+W Media, Inc.

Published by Adams Media, a division of F+W Media, Inc.
57 Littlefield Street, Avon, MA 02322 U.S.A.
www.adamsmedia.com
ISBN 13: 978-1-59337-585-0
ISBN 10: 1-59337-585-9

Printed in the United States of America.

10 9 8 7 6 5

Library of Congress Cataloging-in-Publication Data
Bloch, Jon P.
The everything health guide to adult bipolar disorder : reassuring advice to help you cope / Jon Bloch.
p.   cm. -- (An everything series book)
ISBN 1-59337-585-9
1. Manic-depressive illness--Popular works. 2. Manic-depressive illness--Treatment--Popular
works. 3. Depression, Mental--Popular works. I. Title. II. Series: Everything series.
RC516.B55 2006
616.89'5--dc22
2005033626

All the examples and dialogues used in this book are fictional and have
been created by the author to illustrate disciplinary situations.

Acknowledgments

• • •

Thanks to Kate Burgo at Adams Media, and to my agent, June Clark, at Peter Rubie Literary Agency.

Contents

Introduction

The first question to ask is, what exactly is bipolar disorder? You probably know that it has something to do with "mood swings." But if that was all there was to it, *everyone* would be bipolar, because everyone experiences shifts of mood. A key word to remember about bipolar disorder is *extreme*. It is not just mood swings, but *extreme* mood swings. And "extreme" means "going beyond what is normal or reasonable." People who have bipolar disorder go from a state of *mania*, or extreme high, to *depression*, or extreme low.

Moreover—and this is important—major life events are *not* required to trigger these mood extremes. Someone can shift from high to low (manic to depressed) over seemingly nothing. The shifts themselves can last anywhere from a few minutes to a few months. These manic and depressive moods affect the individual in three important ways: energy level, thought, and behavior.

Energy-wise, someone can seem to be the most high-strung, frenetic person in the world one moment, and the most lethargic and despondent the next. Basic aspects of life that most people take for granted—such as eating, sleeping, getting tired, or feeling refreshed—become major issues for the bipolar person. Given these extreme shifts in energy, it is not surprising that *thought* would likewise be affected. Seemingly from out of nowhere, the bipolar person might decide that everyone is for or against them, and that they themselves are either the greatest person who ever lived—or the worst. Furthermore, since action follows thought, *behavior* becomes erratic and unpredictable. Someone might recklessly quit their job, spend all their money, marry a stranger, or unfairly lash out at a loved one. Taken to an extreme, bipolar behavior can lead to suicide or murder.

Another key word in defining bipolar is *illness*. This might seem too obvious to mention. But both bipolar and non-bipolar people often have difficulty accepting—or remembering—that an "illness" by definition requires treatment. Like any illness, bipolar disorder does not vanish through willpower, or by yelling at someone who has it. It is an illness that at present has no cure. But *treatment* is yet another significant word here, for it is extremely important to understand that bipolar disorder is a *treatable* illness. Many bipolar people can verify that their illness is under control—and that as long as they continue their treatment they live normal, happy, and fulfilling lives.

A final word that is key to understanding bipolar disorder is *episode*. Sometimes, bipolar people experience a perfectly normal hour, day, week, or month. But then will come an hour, day, week, or month of mania or depression—or a volatile mixture of the two. The episodic nature of bipolar disorder is a proverbial double-edged sword. On the one hand, it is a relief to all concerned that the illness does not manifest itself non-stop. But the fact that the symptoms come and go can be confusing, and create false hope that treatment will no longer be needed.

In this book, you hopefully will learn everything you need to know about bipolar disorder: its causes, its symptoms, its treatment, and its history, as well as many other facts and coping tools. But perhaps the main thing to remember is that it *is* treatable. Being bipolar does not have to mean giving up hope for a happy life.

The Basics of Bipolar Disorder

At a fundamental level, bipolar disorder can be defined as: *a treatable illness that is characterized by episodes of extreme mood swings from mania to depression, and affecting the afflicted person's energy level, thoughts, and behavior.* Over two million adults in the United States have been diagnosed as bipolar, and this figure does *not* include bipolar people who have yet to be diagnosed. Consequently, it can be estimated that somewhere between 1 and 5 percent of the U.S. population is bipolar.

History Behind the Disorder

The first known written attempt to recognize and label bipolar disorder came from Aretaeus of Cappadociam in the second century A.D. This pioneering Turk noted the existence of both manic and depressive moods, and even went on to state that they would seem to be related. But it would take over a thousand years before these basic ideas were substantially elaborated upon.

In 1650, a British scientist named Richard Burton wrote a landmark volume entitled, *The Anatomy of Melancholia.* As the title indicates, the focus was on *melancholia,* or what we now call depression. Some of Burton's insights on depression are still employed today. However, given the one-sided emphasis, Burton's model diagnoses patients in terms of their relative "melancholia," under-emphasizing the possible role of mania.

Then in 1854, the Frenchman Jules Falret described *folie circulaire,* or *circular insanity.* He clinically established that suicide and depression could be connected, and furthermore saw a connection between depression and manic states of being—which he asserted was a separate issue from depression by itself. Falret went on to propose a new and distinct psychiatric disorder, *manic-depressive psychosis*, in 1875, and also intimated that there might be genetic factors involved.

At this same time, fellow Frenchman Francois Baillarger gained important insights into the ways in which what we now call bipolar disorder differed from schizophrenia—drawing further attention to bipolar disorder as a distinct and diagnosable state of being. He referred to bipolar disorder as *double insanity*.

It was not until 1913 that the German Emil Krapelin legitimized "manic depressive" as a bona fide terminology through an ambitious study (albeit focusing more on depression than mania). By the early 1930s, Krapelin's ideas on manic depression were the norm within the medical community.

 Fact

"Manic depression" is an older term, but even in some current literature, it is used interchangeably with "bipolar." If you are shopping for information on bipolar disorder and are uncertain about a source that calls it "manic depression," check the publication date. If it has been published within the past ten years, you probably can consider it relatively up-to-date.

In the 1950s and 1960s, an assortment of researchers around the world began conceptualizing a distinction between the *unipolar* (depression) and *bipolar* (mania and depression) along numerous dimensions, including genetics, gender, age when first afflicted, and symptoms. This research led to the 1980 decision by the American Psychiatric Association to refer to the body of symptoms as "bipolar disorder" in its official *Diagnostic and Statistical Manual*.

Bipolar I Versus Bipolar II

Bipolar disorder takes several different forms. One helpful distinction to remember is that some people tend to experience more intense mania, and some people tend to experience more intense depression. This basic difference means two main varieties of the illness: Bipolar I and Bipolar II.

Bipolar I

Bipolar I disorder is considered the most serious form of the illness. It features three basic types of episodes: manic and/or manic-depressive episodes (also called *mixed episodes*), and at least one depressive episode. Sometimes both mania and depression are present at more or less the same time. But the emphasis is somewhat more on mania. There are usually several manic episodes and/or manic-depressive ones, and then at least one depressive one. The manic side tends to be present more often, and/or more intense while it is present.

However, in emphasizing the manic side, the depressive side should not be trivialized. If mania is more likely to lead to spontaneous harm to self or others, depression is more likely to lead to suicide. Mania can fuel intense anger or mistrust. Depression can make people feel so bad about life that out of "mercy" they decide to kill other people. Since depression tends to limit one's energy, the murder victims are often children—as children are relatively easy to contain, especially if they are one's own.

It is not difficult to see why it is essential that the person with Bipolar I seek treatment; if untreated, the person will be lucky to be hospitalized before causing major harm. In fact, someone who is having an untreated Bipolar I episode is quite likely to seem like someone who *should* be hospitalized for his own good.

Bipolar II

Bipolar II is characterized by depressive episodes similar to Bipolar I, and, again, there tend to be more manic episodes. However, Bipolar II includes manic episodes that are less intense, called hypomanic episodes. Thus, while Bipolar II is not as serious as Bipolar I, it can be harder to detect. This is problematic in several ways.

 ## Question

What is Bipolar III?
A controversial diagnosis, this is what happens when someone is diagnosed for depression, and the prescribed medication seems to produce manic or hypomanic symptoms. Thus, Bipolar III is perceived to be a "man-made" condition that results only from the medication for depression. Nonetheless, it must be treated as extremely serious, as it can result in many of the same consequences as other manifestations of mania.

First, it often means a lack of proper treatment. If being treated only for depression, the Bipolar II individual simply is not getting full treatment.

Next, there is a risk that symptoms may escalate. While it is possible to stay at the Bipolar II level indefinitely, it is also possible that it will escalate into Bipolar I. And this becomes more likely over time as life events exacerbate the untreated symptoms.

Additionally, there is the matter of heightened depression. Since the episodes of depression are more powerful than the lesser hypomanic ones, thoughts of death and suicide have the potential to be all the more heightened. The seemingly "happy" person who much to everyone's surprise commits suicide might well have been suffering from undiagnosed Bipolar II.

Manic Episodes

Some people think that simply being a high-energy person is the same thing as being manic—but it is not. There is a profound contrast between having high energy and having bipolar disorder. And there are easy ways of telling the difference.

Rapid Speech, High Energy, and Euphoria

First, bipolar people experience lightning-quick ideas that they can barely verbalize fast enough. Yet verbalize them they will; people experiencing this type of acceleration will talk non-stop. Their speech may even start to sound like nonsense—rhyming words for no reason, or making hard-to-follow observations that resemble the heightened perceptions some people experience from recreational drugs. The speed of the speech can be too fast to follow, and the speaker often develops a hoarse voice from talking so much.

Another common symptom is seemingly boundless energy. These people might go for days without sleep. At the same time, they exhibit a childlike blend of fascination and impatience toward different activities or people. Like a child quickly engaged—and just as quickly bored—the manic bipolar person flits from one pursuit to the next.

L., Essential

Bipolar disorder frequently plays a role in serious crimes. About 25 percent of people hospitalized for mental disorder commit a violent crime within two weeks of being committed. Recent studies suggest significant connections between bipolar disorder and spousal and child abuse. Mania can inspire people to commit acts of larceny, extortion, or fraud.

Not surprisingly, mania can also be characterized by a strong sense of euphoria—but this euphoria can switch to anger or hostility in an instant. Someone who one moment seems deliriously happy seems irritated by the smallest thing the next.

Manic Thinking, Manic Psychosis

Manic episodes also involve *manic thinking*, or grandiosity—believing that you are much more than you are. The slightest self-accomplishment is elevated; taking out the garbage might be talked about as if having found a cure for cancer. An individual seems all about self-confidence, and is dangerously optimistic. Nothing bad could possibly happen to the "Great Me." Insight and self-reflection take a back seat to denial. Nothing that one has ever said or done could possibly be less than perfection. Because constructive self-criticism is not an option, it can be extremely difficult to point out to the afflicted person that something is wrong.

Left unchecked, this manic thinking can achieve the level of *manic psychosis*, in which people might hallucinate or hear voices that support this grandiose view of self. Common delusions include having more talent or skill than one actually possesses, or an exaggerated air of wealth or aristocracy. Some might even decide they can heal the sick by their touch. Yet these same delusions can also inspire a sense of persecution—that this great self is so envied by others that it is being unfairly attacked or plotted against.

Risk-taking, Sex, and Nosiness

Accelerated psychomotor activity can also inspire risk-taking behavior. This can include: sudden and unplanned trips, business investments, and even marriage; compulsive gambling; giving away possessions or paying people's bills; running up huge phone bills; buying expensive cars, jewelry, or large quantities of less expensive items; and calling attention to oneself in public by shouting, preaching, dancing, or singing in the street.

Sexually speaking, mania creates an intensely increased appetite. Someone might inappropriately become involved or uninvolved with an intimate partner for some sudden and intense sexual need. Not uncommonly, these individuals have a long list of marriages, or people with whom they have been sexual.

Yet another common symptom of a manic episode is inappropriate involvement in other people's lives—being a super-busybody. Personal or professional matters that are none of this person's business are suddenly treated as though they were. Bipolar people might make phone calls at inappropriate times, offer long-winded and unsolicited advice, or make bullying threats. Friends and family often distance themselves to escape this meddlesome behavior.

 Fact

> Jayson Blair's career as a *New York Times* reporter came to an abrupt halt in 2003 when it was learned that he copied stories from other newspapers, and fabricated quotes and sources. Apparently, Blair has been diagnosed as bipolar. Grandiosity, inflated self-esteem, and high-risk behavior all seem to have played a role in his unfortunate self-destruction as a journalist.

Not surprisingly, a manic episode can require hospitalization, for the safety of both the patient and those around him or her. Otherwise, it can lead to tragic consequences.

Depressive Episodes

In many ways, the depression experienced by the bipolar individual is indeed the polar opposite of mania—and can also be extremely dangerous. There is a shutting down of the senses; one seems to notice or experience very little, and seems barely alive. Instead of feeling grandiose, the bipolar person now feels guilty and worthless.

Reverse of Mania

Eating and sleeping patterns are reversed. If in the manic state they could not slow down to eat, bipolar people will now be ravenously hungry. (Or, if in the manic state they took great pleasure in eating, they now will have a loss of appetite.) Rather than having so much energy that they can go without sleep, they now appear to have no energy at all, and will want to do little besides sleep. Also not uncommon are sudden complaints about aches and pains that do not have any traceable origin.

In an episode of depression, activities that used to engage the person no longer do. It becomes hard to concentrate on anything at all; gone is the intense (if fleeting) interest of the manic episode. Likewise, the depressed bipolar individual seems to lose engagement in people that he formerly cared about. The afflicted individual becomes reclusive, turning down social invitations, and virtually not wanting to see anybody.

Depressed bipolar people feel very easily defeated. Nothing seems worth trying, because whatever it is, the individual is convinced it will not work out. Listless and lethargic, these people seem uninterested in everything, and have difficulty making decisions about even the smallest things.

Depression and Suicide

Like manic episodes, depression can involve anger and irritability. But this does not fluctuate with euphoria—instead, it fluctuates with anxiety, fear, and agitation. The bipolar individual might cry for long periods, and for seemingly no reason. Even when not crying, these people seem to carry a grave sadness about them.

L Essential

Manic episodes feature what is called accelerated psychomotor activity. This means that there is an increase in rapid bodily activity that is triggered by mental changes. By contrast, depressive episodes are typified by psychomotor retardation. The body is less rapid and active, due to a diminishing of mental activity.

At its most extreme, a depressive episode can lead to thoughts of suicide. Life seems so not worth living—and so painful—and one feels so unworthy, that dying might seem the one viable option. (See also Chapter 8.)

Even short of a suicide attempt, depressed bipolar people will feel a strong attraction to matters pertaining to death. Ironically, it might be the one topic that sparks their interest. In fact, sometimes these highly depressed people will seem strangely energized before taking their own lives. Others might even think that the person was "getting better" or "snapping out of it" and are extremely shocked to learn that this person committed suicide. Fascination with death, combined with the relief in believing the pain of living will soon end, is often mistaken for improvement.

Hypomania

The relatively minor manic episodes seen in Bipolar II are called hypomanic. Essentially, many of the same areas are affected as in mania, but the difference is in degree.

Instead of feeling utterly euphoric, the person having a hypo-manic episode experiences "only" heightened confidence. With hypomania, you probably would *not* feel that nothing bad at all could happen to you. But you might notice how assertive or outgoing you suddenly are—or that you have the nerve to ride a scary roller coaster, or sing karaoke, when moments ago you did not. You feel oddly in tune with life and feel like you know just what to say or do.

There is likely to be more sexual activity, and more thoughtless spending with hypomania. Yet once again, none of this is quite at the same danger level as mania. For example, people might be more dis-creet in pursuing sex, and more likely to spend too much to pay all their bills that month, as opposed to spending *everything* they have. And unlike mania, hypomania is not associated with full-blown psychosis.

In hypomania, people usually cannot do without sleep altogether, but they do sleep *less*. Their thoughts are not a total gibberish of non-stop stream of consciousness, but thoughts are heightened and more rapid than usual. Likewise, hypomanics do not talk non-stop until they are hoarse, but they do talk more than usual. For example, people who normally do not interrupt others when they are talking now suddenly are unable to resist doing so. Perhaps these people even apologize for talking so much, while privately wondering why they are being such chatterboxes.

Puzzling Mood Shifts

In hypomania, sudden confidence can just as suddenly leave. People who met you while you were being the proverbial "life of the party" might be baffled at the relative level of social discomfort you display once back to "normal." On the other hand, people who have known you longer might have wondered why suddenly you were not behaving like your regular self. They mistakenly might have thought the "new" self was an improvement, or it might have made them uncomfortable, but in either case those closest to you will notice a change.

People might be exasperated by the hypomanic's ebb and flow of confidence and drive—including the hypomanic. Undiagnosed hypomanics might wonder why they could not stand up to their boss on Friday when they had no trouble doing so on Monday. Over time, the cycle renders people all the more confused about themselves, and all the more apprehensive about these unexplainable shifts of personality.

Concentration and Goals

Hypomania sees individuals becoming quite easily distracted, and having difficulty concentrating. But once again, it is not as dramatic as in full-scale mania. For example, rather than absolutely dropping one activity (or person) for the next, it might be that someone complains of having trouble concentrating on a project. In conversation with a hypomanic person, you might often be asked to repeat what you just said, because the other person was thinking of something else.

Yet for all the fairly rapid changes and distractions that accompany hypomania, the afflicted individual might be obsessed with achieving a goal. It can be a personal or professional goal, but probably the Bipolar II person will talk about it frequently. Decisions might even be made surrounding this goal. For example, someone might turn down an invitation to go out to dinner because a work report "must" get finished, even though it is not due yet. In reality, little time that evening might actually get spent working on whatever it is. *Or* there might be an extremely intense focus upon the minutest details, doing more than is necessary. Perhaps a five-page report becomes twenty-five pages. It is as if you are not only scrubbing the floor with a toothbrush, but *enjoying* it. People who have abused diet pills and amphetamines sometimes experience this type of single-minded focus that may or may not withstand the threat of distraction.

Dangers of Hypomania

Though more manic than someone's "normal" behavior, hypo-manic episodes are less likely to signal that the individual in question needs hospitalization, or is otherwise in serious danger. In fact, some might think that being hypomanic might not be so bad. It has its obvious drawbacks, yet it also might sound attractive to feel highly confident, or be goal-driven. It even sometimes passes for "normal."

Essential

There are articles in business journals in which an author claims that employers should go out of their way to hire hypomanic people, that everyone should strive to be hypomanic, or that hypomanic people are happier. This ironic reverse discrimination shows that many people see only the superficial, "up" side of hypomania, and not the depression or other serious problems.

However, there is an irony in Bipolar II: Since hypomania is less likely to cause serious problems in someone's everyday life, an individual may be misdiagnosed as simply depressed. The hypomanic state might seem to be enthusiasm, and is not recognized as part of the problem. But it is extremely important to remember that hypomania *is* related to depression and *is* part of the same illness. Where there is hypomania, *there will be depression.*

Cylclothymia and Hyperthymia

If you have a basic grasp of the manic, depressive, and hypomanic episodes that comprise Bipolar I and Bipolar II, you already know quite a lot about bipolar disorder. But there are two other illnesses that feature relatively minor symptoms of bipolar disorder: cyclothymia and hyperthymia. There are differing opinions in the medical community as to whether these are minor versions of bipolar disorder, or similar but different disorders.

Cylclothymia

Cyclothymia is characterized by less intense cycles of *both* mania and depression. (By contrast, Bipolar II is milder *only* when it comes to mania.) Left untreated, cyclothymia can lead to full-blown bipolar disorder.

The manic symptoms are similar to hypomania: dramatic shifts from high to low energy, unpredictable mood changes, marked changes in ability to concentrate or engage the self, and heightened or dulled perceptions. Emotions are experienced with intensity, and there is a desire to shock or be outrageous. However, there is not necessarily an exceptionally powerful sexual urge. Though the depression is not as intense as in Bipolar I or II, the individual with cyclothymia will still feel quite depressed.

On balance, cyclothymia, though less dramatic than Bipolar I or II, will significantly impair one's ability to succeed and find happiness. It absolutely must be treated, especially since it can intensify into something more serious.

Hyperthymia

Hyperthymia is a state associated with high activity and inflated self-esteem. In many ways, it is like having nothing but hypomania. But a crucial difference is that hyperthymia is *not* episodic. Instead, it is experienced habitually, or long-term. It is somewhat like being on a "permanent high." This might sound appealing, but it can cause serious problems. Like any "high," it tends to render the individual less than fully grounded in the present moment. And as with other bipolar manifestations, hyperthymia is often associated with sleeping problems, having an inappropriately high sex drive, and being overly involved in other people's business.

 ## Fact

On occasion, a patient seems unmistakably bipolar, yet does not seem to fit any of the known patterns. In these instances, someone might be diagnosed as having bipolar disorder not otherwise specified, or Bipolar NOS. This classification enables a doctor to consider the patient bipolar, and thus see how the illness is or is not being manifested according to classic diagnosis and symptoms.

On the surface of things, people with hyperthymia seem optimistic and full of energy. They radiate self-confidence and are self-reliant; they seem to believe they can do whatever needs to be done. They also are not afraid to be where the action is—they thrive on new experiences that promise variety, intrigue, and novelty. Usually, they have a great many personal interests, as well as plans for the future. Hyperthymic people are also articulate and witty.

 ## Alert

Like hypomania, hyperthymia is sometimes misconstrued as a wholly positive condition. There are people who say they wish they were hyperthymic, or that they are "almost as happy as a hyperthymic." But what goes up must inevitably come down, and despite the seemingly constant high, hyperthymia does make people vulnerable to depression. Additionally, hyperthymic people can alienate or annoy other people for their inability to experience certain kinds of feelings.

Remember, though, that these people are *habitually* these things; it is not about feeling upbeat based on one's quality of life, but a physiological limitation. People accused of not having a "soul"—of missing some vital human emotion—might be hyperthymic. They stay busy and self-involved, yet some healthy response to the full range of life experience seems to elude them.

For example, let us say that your father just died, and one of your brothers seems to have no reaction. He just keeps on being his usual busy and upbeat self. There are numerous explanations for this: maybe he grieves privately, is in denial, or is afraid to show much feeling around others. But it is also possible that the appropriate grief simply does not register with him because he is hyperthymic.

Other Variations

In addition to cyclothymia and hyperthymia, there are a few other kinds of episodes that have been characterized as belonging to bipolar disorder. These include: mixed episodes, rapid cycling, and mixed mania.

Mixed Episodes

A manic-depressive or mixed episode often occurs in Bipolar I. The mania and depression occur at the same time, as part of the same misadventure. For example, rather than being euphoric for days or weeks before becoming filled with despair for days or weeks, one is euphoric for perhaps just a matter of minutes before becoming riddled with despair—only to be euphoric again a few minutes later.

Mixed episodes can be especially confusing to the onlooker who does not know about someone's bipolar history. It is all too easy to lose patience with someone having a mixed episode, because it seems no matter what you say or do it makes someone unhappy—or else fails to calm her down.

Rapid Cycling

Rapid cycling means that a patient experiences episodes at least four times a year, each cycle lasting for a relatively short time. In extreme cases, some people rapid cycle several times a day. All told, approximately 20 percent of bipolar patients experience rapid cycling. It is associated more often with Bipolar II than Bipolar I, but it can also occur in Bipolar I. It is also associated with mixed episodes, and with bipolar children.

This rapid cycling usually begins with an episode of depression. It happens more to women than men. It also is more associated with a given patient's first few years of being bipolar. Some research further suggests that it might be more common in bipolar patients who are also diagnosed as mentally retarded. Additionally, it might be related to thyroid problems, or substance abuse.

Mixed Mania

Mixed mania is a combination of depressive and hypo- to manic conditions present at the same time. It is rather like having nothing but mixed episodes. For example, the individual might feel simultaneously grandiose *and* suicidal. This affliction is also sometimes called *dysphoric mania.*

Like a child who inherits the worst features of the parents, mixed mania manifests many of the most dangerous traits associated with mania (or hypomania) and depression. The person in this state of illness often cannot sleep, is depressed and suicidal, and experiences delusions of persecution. She is easily excited and grandiose—yet is also easy to panic, easy to anger, and highly agitated. Given both the high energy level and depression, the individual might plot an elaborate suicide that requires a great deal of planning.

Anhedonia, or an inability to enjoy life, often logically accompanies this death wish. The thought of staying alive fills these people with dread, because all they can think of is all that is likely to go wrong, and everything that will hurt or frighten them.

CHAPTER 2

How Do You Know
If You're Bipolar?

Everyone experiences ups and downs—within a day, week, month, year, or lifetime. But how "up" or "down" you feel might be heavily influenced by forces beyond your control. For example, how "up" could you possibly feel if something tragic just happened to you? How, then, can you tell if your ups and downs fall within a seemingly normal range, or if they signal the presence of a serious mood disorder such as bipolar? The information in this chapter will help you decide.

Mistaking Bipolar for "Normal"

Ironically, though more is known about bipolar disorder today than ever before, the frantic way of life in today's world can make it harder to tell if someone is bipolar. Today, we do not just admire achievement, but overachievement. Whatever someone does, she should do more of it, and do it better. Hence, the manic side of bipolar disorder might fit all too well with someone's career or lifestyle.

People might marvel at how much a bipolar individual accomplishes, and wonder where all that energy comes from. But then, when the mania slides over to depression, people might chalk it up to "working too hard"—which leads to the conclusion that all that is needed is a little rest. Or people might wonder why this highly motivated person is so profoundly plagued with self-doubt. Maybe they will conclude that insecurity is a good thing, because it makes you push yourself harder.

Fact

U.S. rates for bipolar disorder are higher than in many other countries; for example, about 33 percent higher than Canada, and close
to 50 percent higher than Germany. It is interesting to speculate as
to why this is. Could our high-pressure way of life be a factor? Do we
test people more often for bipolar, or do we use different testing
criteria altogether?

In still other situations, such an individual might suddenly turn
on close associates or loved ones. People might decide that this person has one of those "larger than life" personalities. Like others who
are very driven to succeed, this is someone who is easier to admire
from a safe distance.

Essential

Bipolar disorder should not be thought of as "romantic" or "interesting." If you find yourself saying, "He is probably bipolar, but for him
it's a good thing, because it helps him accomplish so much more,"
there is something fundamental about bipolar disorder that you do
not understand. It is essential that bipolar disorder be viewed as a
serious condition requiring treatment.

However successful a bipolar person might be, treatment is still
essential. The mania is still destined to get out of control, and this
seemingly successful person might well end up making tragically
unfortunate choices. Also, the depressive part of the cycle will appear,
and the great success will turn mysteriously despondent. When
someone who seems to have "everything" mysteriously commits

suicide—or, short of that, suddenly loses it all in a strange urge to self-destruct—it is possible that this is someone who is bipolar but does not know it. He may actually need diagnosis and treatment.

General Warning Signs

Bipolar behavior is human behavior. Although it is extreme, non-bipolar people might from time to time exhibit similar characteristics. Crisis situations, major life changes, and so-called recreational drug use are some of the scenarios in which someone might seem to manifest some of these qualities. Therefore, the presence of certain thoughts and behaviors does not automatically mean that someone is bipolar. There can be other explanations. Still, it is extremely useful to be aware of certain bipolar warning signs.

- **Sudden changes in behavior:** These can include changes in eating and sleeping patterns, as well as energy level and confidence in personal or professional activities.
- **Poor concentration skills:** The person either never finishes anything, or else overdoes it. Also, an individual might stay up all night working on something, only to destroy it come morning— as if to create and destroy were one and the same process.
- **Extreme arrogance:** The individual might talk about nothing but herself, and always in the most superlative of terms. Praise is always expected—even for feats of questionable value. There might be fabrications about past achievements, family history, or even spiritual matters.
- **Inappropriate anger:** If nothing in a situation seems to warrant anger, and the anger turns to an extreme expression of rage, there is cause for concern. This is especially true if property gets destroyed.
- **Excessive meddling:** Someone who is extremely intent on telling other people what to do, cannot stop thinking about what other people should do, and spends an inordinate amount of

time talking about other people behind their backs might be bipolar.

- **Sexual compulsion:** A bipolar person often makes inappropriate sexual advances toward others, or takes dangerous risks, destroys personal relations, moves in with strangers, or destroys finances in order to have sex.
- **Imaginary aches and pains:** If someone experiences bouts of body aches and complaints that more than one doctor cannot find any cause for, it is wise to delve further into the person's thought and behavioral patterns.
- **Inappropriate risk-taking:** Some bipolar people engage in dangerous relationships, financial ventures, dishonesty, law-breaking, or physical activities to fulfill a self-destructive desire for excitement.

At the most obvious level, someone who has previously been diagnosed bipolar but never did anything about it is likely to be headed for a bipolar episode. Similarly, someone whom a doctor encouraged to be tested for bipolar disorder and never did so might in fact *be* bipolar, and therefore experience dangerous mood swings.

 Alert

Though treatment of bipolar disease costs society, not treating it is even more expensive. While about $8 billion is spent each year on treatment, about $40 billion is wasted due to lost wages and compensation, suicide, and lost productivity to family members who must function as caregivers to bipolar people unable to take care of themselves.

There also appears to be a genetic component to bipolar disorder. Someone who has had a family member diagnosed as depressed or bipolar might also be bipolar. If no one was formally diagnosed, there still may have been a parent, elder, or sibling who was danger-ous, or at least extremely hard to be around, because of extreme mood fluctuations.

Behavioral Extremes and Private Thoughts

Behavioral extremes are strong indications that a person is bipolar. If you—or someone you know—exhibit extreme behavior, you are advised to see a doctor. You are not necessarily bipolar, but there is no harm or shame in finding out—and only good can come from it. Some more common behavioral extremes include:

- **Busy bee/slug:** Person who is always either doing many things at once, or else is utterly listless and lethargic.
- **Life of the party/recluse:** Person who tends to either be the charismatic center of attention, or else cannot wait to unplug the phone and stay away from everyone.
- **Chatterbox/silent type:** Person who either cannot shut up, or else never says anything.
- **Optimist/pessimist:** Person who either acts like he's on top of the world, or else seems to finds nothing good in life at all. In the optimistic phase, there is often a strong belief in supersti-tion or mystical pre-destiny. Then, in the downward swing to pessimism, life seems utterly meaningless and chaotic—or else fated to bring ruin to the self.

While external behaviors are often signs of being bipolar, internal thoughts can also indicate the disorder. Much like behaviors, private thoughts also tend to gravitate toward the extremes.

- **"I am happy, confident, and loved." / "I am sad, frightened, and alone."** Someone might be euphoric one moment, depressed the next. Such a person feels utterly at ease and secure, or else anxious and frightened.

- **"I feel things too strongly." / "I never feel much of anything."** A person may either feel that she is the only person in the room (or in the family, or on the face of the earth) who has deep, honest emotional responses—or else she believes she is the least emotional person.
- **"I am better than other people." / "I am worse than other people."** There are individuals who either feel bored by everyone and vastly superior, or else feel utterly unworthy of anyone's companionship. Often these people seem most eager to make friends at first, but then become extremely critical or short-tempered.
- **"I love life." / "I hate life."** Some people either feel swept up in a dizzy waltz of rapture, or else think that everything is useless, meaningless—or even foolish, ugly, and distorted. At either extreme, there might be voices or hallucinations. At the depressive extreme, the person wants to commit suicide.

If you are concerned that someone you know might be bipolar, you can encourage this person to see a doctor, or at least read up on the topic. More information will be provided later on how you might try to do this as tactfully as possible. Of course, identifying the symptoms of bipolar disorder in the self can be an equally or even more tricky matter. People are more likely to notice the symptoms after being treated—medication makes the contrast between symptomatic and non-symptomatic behavior much clearer. The sad irony here is that the untreated patient is more likely to believe nothing is wrong—or that nothing can be done to help.

See a Doctor

If there is a possibility that you or someone you care about is bipolar, the only way to be certain is to see a doctor. You can start by visiting your general practitioner (GP). Even if your GP decides you are bipolar and prescribes medication, you should always get a second opinion from a psychiatrist. A general practitioner is good for diagnosing more common ailments, but should be referring you to a psychiatrist if there is a possibility that you have a serious mental condition.

 Alert

Do not confuse a psychologist with a psychiatrist. Many maladies are helped through psychology. But if there is a possibility that the true nature of your problem is an actual mental illness such as bipolar disorder, only a medical doctor can diagnose this and prescribe medication.

Psychologists address mental and emotional problems from the standpoint of life experience. The goal is to get you to think and feel differently about yourself so that you can live your daily life in more productive ways. They are doctors of philosophy, and so have the title of Ph.D. However, psychiatrists are medical doctors, and so have the title of M.D. or D.O.

Diagnosis

To some extent, doctors are at the mercy of patients when making a diagnosis; they can only speculate on what else might be true if you tell them only half the story. So, do not be afraid, and do not be ashamed—answer every question fully and honestly. Research is under way to develop a means of genetically testing for bipolar disorder. But in the meantime, honest self-reports given to a medical doctor are the principle means of diagnosis. Your doctor will ask you to describe your energy, thoughts, and behavioral patterns, and also ask a series of specific questions. One or more standardized tests might be used in the process.

Ideally, a doctor correctly diagnoses patients all of the time, but even if they get it right only *most* of the time, obviously people should still see doctors. But you should have an informed, pro-active stance as a medical patient. Probably your doctor does know best, but you should still ask questions.

Essential

Bipolar disorder diagnosis requires patience on the part of both the patient and doctor. At present, only about 20 percent of patients receive a full diagnosis in a year or less. While it can be frustrating to have to try different treatments or re-check for symptoms, it shows that generally psychiatrists are not casual in diagnosing people as having serious mood disorders.

Be a Good Patient

As a patient, there are two personas you want to avoid. First, there is the eager-to-please patient who tries to second-guess what the doctor wants to hear in order to provide it. For example, the patient might be asked how things have been going, and give a knee-jerk response of "fine." This patient so wants the doctor to be right that even if some aspects of the treatment are not working, the patient does not say this. If a doctor lets slip that she is predicting a certain response from the treatment, the patient might report confirmation of it even if such was not the case.

On the other hand, the rebellious patient might insist that *nothing* is going well even if this is not true. Patients often rebel against treatment when they feel they are being forced to see a doctor, or when the patient does not really want to get better. The rebellious patient will scrupulously avoid mentioning certain things, or else talk about them in a way that makes them seem more or less important than they are. The overriding theme will be that the treatment is not working—which is to say the doctor does not know how to properly connect to the patient, and/or that no one in the world can.

A responsible psychiatrist will not make a diagnosis of bipolar (or anything else) simply for the sake of making a diagnosis; she will relay only what the data signal. Thus, it is hoped that once given medication, you will notice a positive difference. However, if you feel no different—or feel worse—you need to be honest with your doctor, and speak up about that, too. Diagnosis is a collaborative process between doctor and patient. It is your mental health at stake; do not be passive about it.

Get a Second Opinion

Being treated for bipolar disorder is a lifetime proposition, so you owe it to yourself to seek out a second opinion. This is especially important if the medication you are taking does not seem to be doing what it is supposed to do. The same holds true in reverse. If your first doctor says you are not bipolar but you still think you might be, see what a second doctor has to say.

Beware of Misdiagnosis

When it comes to misdiagnosis of bipolar disorder, the most common errors are: confusing one type of bipolar for another and checking only for depression. If you are being tested for depression by a psychiatrist, you should ask if the doctor is also considering the possibility of mania. If you are diagnosed with a form of bipolar disorder, you should ask which type it is. It also is in your best interests to seek a second opinion if at all possible.

If you start a regimen of treatment you should find out all you can about the medication you are taking. A good doctor will answer all of your questions, but you can also use resources such as the Internet to find out even more. Once on medication, you need to be scrupulously honest with the doctor—and with yourself—as to what is or is not changing, and in what way.

Don't Let Limitations Stop You

Money can be a major limitation—some people have no health insurance, or their insurance will only pay for some of their needs. But no matter how delicate your financial situation, it is worthwhile to pursue a first and second opinion, a sound diagnosis, and, if necessary, treatment. If you live in a relatively small community, and do not have access to a variety of psychiatrists, then see one in the next town over—or in the nearest big city. Your mental well-being is more important than inconvenience or spending a few extra dollars.

What if you get that second opinion and the second psychiatrist makes a contradictory diagnosis? In this case, you might want to consider the specificity of the differing opinions, and ask as many questions as possible of both sources. You can also compare the two doctors along dimensions such as years of experience, references from other patients, and how well each seems to understand you and is willing to listen to you. If you're still in doubt, seek out a third opinion.

 Fact

According to the Depression and Bipolar Support Alliance (DPSA), 87 percent of the treated patients report being satisfied with the care they receive from their doctors. Despite the fact that diagnosis can be a drawn-out process, patients seem to be generally pleased with how they are treated—both in terms of their illnesses, and as human beings.

Once you're on medication, stay on it! No matter how stable your moods have become, you will need to keep taking the medication. You moods are stable *because of* the medication, so if you stop taking it the mood swings of earlier times *will* return.

Evolving Knowledge of Bipolar Disorder

Let's say that you are told two different things about bipolar disorder from two different, seemingly reliable sources. Which should you believe? Is one automatically "true," and the other "false?" The answer is not so simple.

Science is an emergent, evolving process. Scientists do not suddenly know "everything" about whatever it is they are studying. Instead, new information is constantly built upon the existing foundation of knowledge. Sometimes new findings even call into question the present day assumptions. Likewise, the collective knowledge about bipolar disorder keeps growing over time; and like any other scientific endeavor, sometimes there are even disagreements about it. But on balance, there is much that *is* agreed upon. People with bipolar disorder can consider themselves relatively fortunate to be diagnosed in today's world, when so much is known about cause, symptoms, and treatment.

Important Trends

Three important historical trends helped achieve today's state of knowledge on bipolar disorder. First, in the 1790s, Phillippe Pinel radically altered the treatment of the mentally ill by asserting that liberal and humane therapy was needed, as opposed to punishing, physical torture (which had been the trend for centuries). This set in motion the widespread belief that patients with mental conditions could respond positively to certain kinds of treatment aimed at improvement.

Then, about a hundred years later, Sigmund Freud ushered in the era of psychotherapy. Freud sought purely psychological explanations for mental afflictions—which does not apply to bipolar disorder, since it does have a strong biological component. Nonetheless, the Freudian tradition of the talking patient helps psychiatrists in today's world to likewise elicit a sense of which thoughts and behaviors are problematic, and to diagnose accordingly.

Finally, in the 1950s, the era of pharmacological treatment for mental illness was ushered in—rapidly diminishing the number of people who were hospitalized for mental disorders. Medications would see many refinements over the ensuing decades, but the essential notion that bipolar disorder could be treated by the right combination of chemicals radically altered the medical community's response.

Why Is There Not Yet a Cure?

Even after the previous explanation, you might still be wondering: If we can put a man on the moon, why can we not find a cure for mental illnesses such as bipolar disorder?

One reason is that research is expensive—and only so much public and private funding to date has been acquired. Bipolar disorder causes death and destruction as surely as done any illness, but because its symptoms are often seen as "only" mental, it is not always viewed as urgent a matter as other kinds of afflictions.

Ⅼ. Essential

One of the most outspoken advocates for education on bipolar disorder is the openly bipolar actress, Patty Duke. In her autobiography, *Call Me Anna*, she writes frankly about the extreme mood swings that hampered her life until being diagnosed. She provides the reader with an accurate picture of what it is like to live with untreated bipolar disorder.

But even if funding were not an issue, it is important to remember that the research community sometimes comes to slightly different conclusions about the meaning of different factors. For example, some have argued that Bipolar I and II should be considered two separate illnesses. "Cyclothymia" now refers to more minor mood swings, but for a time in the 1800s it was used to describe the entire spectrum of conditions.

Such disagreements are healthy, in that they keep the research on bipolar as honest as possible, and also keep the proverbial door open to new findings. Maybe someday everything *will* be known about bipolar disorder. But in the meantime it is a work in progress. Thus, if one book or doctor offers *slightly* different information about the nature or causes of bipolar disorder, you need not be overly concerned. Just be aware that there sometimes are differences of opinion, and understand that these differences probably exist for good reason.

Comparing Bipolar to Other Mood Disorders

Part of the process of diagnosis is determining if you are bipolar, or if you have another condition. Even if you have fairly strong mood swings, you may not be bipolar. There are a number of other mood disorders that exhibit symptoms similar to those of bipolar disorder, a situation that often leads to misdiagnosis. These various other disorders can also be quite serious for the afflicted person and/or her loved ones.

Varieties of Mood Disorders

If you think you may have bipolar disorder, it is important to know about some other mood disorders to compare and contrast symptoms. There are several different diagnoses that are possible in this situation. One possibility, of course, is that you do not have a mood disorder, and that your problem is something else. Perhaps you need to see a psychologist, and work on your issues in other kinds of ways. Another possibility is that you are not bipolar and have some other mood disorder altogether. Thirdly, you might be diagnosed as bipolar, in which case you should begin serious treatment at once. A fourth possibility is a mixed diagnosis—you are told you are bipolar and have one or more other mood disorders. If you are given a mixed diagnosis, you should have it explained to you why you are both (or all three or four) of these things: what symptoms do you have that cannot be explained by only one of these disorders?

Many mood disorders can be highly problematic, but bipolar disorder is often regarded as the most serious kind of mood disorder. It can present the most dangerous and pervasive symptoms—

including outright hallucinations. However, the presence of other mood disorders can complicate bipolar disorder in several ways.

Fact

Recreational drug use—and abuse—often results in symptoms similar to those of bipolar disorder. Recreational drugs fall into three main categories: stimulants, including cocaine, crack cocaine, and amphetamines; depressants, such as alcohol, tranquilizers, and barbiturates; and hallucinogens, like LSD.

First, other mood disorders can exacerbate bipolar. The symptoms associated with a given disorder might serve to trigger a manic or depressive episode. Also, other mood disorders can make it harder to treat bipolar disorder. If another mood disorder also requires medication, it might not be compatible with medication for bipolar disorder. Finally, other mood disorders can make it more difficult to detect bipolar disorder. Some of the symptoms of other mood disorders resemble some of the symptoms of bipolar disorder, and so making a thorough diagnosis can be that much more challenging.

Borderline Personality Disorder (BPD)

BPD is possibly the most serious of the non-bipolar disorders. It derived its name from the belief that it was a borderline psychosis. Now, however, it is often thought to be treatable through cognitive therapy—that it is not so much a biochemical disorder but a trained inability to regulate one's emotions. However, BPD can be co-present with bipolar disorder, and heighten some of its symptoms.

Unstable Moods

BPD features instability of mood and behavior, which in turn makes for an insecure personal and professional life, as well as a rickety self-image. Someone might abruptly quit a job, end a relationship, or make an enemy out of a friend due to a sudden switch of mood. When the proverbial dust settles and things return to "normal," the person with BPD might be as mystified as everyone else concerned as to exactly what just happened.

People with BPD suffer severe anger, anxiety, and depression, but the symptoms usually last only a matter of minutes or hours, and seldom beyond a day. While the symptoms last, however, the individual can cause considerable damage to herself or others. An episode of BPD focuses on aggressive impulses, which can be expressed through anger toward others, injury to self, substance abuse, binge eating or spending, or high-risk sex. Temporarily warped perceptions can cause people to impulsively abandon otherwise productive goals or endeavors. Despite a certain air of superiority during these episodes, they can feel unworthy of happiness. Much of their anger is self-directed, and can involve self-injury or even a suicide attempt.

Though reactions can be more extreme than the situation warrants, they are not the result of physiological change so much as a psychological response. While bipolar disorder can involve mood changes literally over nothing, with BPD there is *some* tangible cause for the change of mood. If the situation resolves itself, the moodiness might instantly disappear. In the eyes of the person with BPD, you can be the greatest human being of all time one moment, and the worst the next.

Since the person returns to "normal" after these relatively short episodes, BPD often goes undiagnosed. BPD people—and those around them—might mistakenly assume that it is simply a matter of having a bad day. A BPD person is likely to be regarded as someone who would be okay if only he did not get "that way" sometimes.

Poor Social Skills

BPD people feel very easily abandoned, and are extremely sensitive to rejection. At the slightest slight, they go from thinking someone or something is just what they have been looking for to feeling betrayed, and angrily deciding that they have been wasting their time. Not surprisingly, relationships tend to be unstable, and riddled with conflict.

Such people can feel frustrated over being misunderstood. When their bad moods are over, they are so over that the BPD individual can scarcely even remember them. When the other person involved in the conflict tends to avoid her afterward, the BPD person might express genuine perplexity. She does not understand what the "big deal" is, since she is no longer angry.

Essential

People with BPD have difficulty coping with boredom. They cannot last long at a repetitive job, and on a personal level can equate boredom with cruelty—as though someone were intentionally plotting to hurt their feelings by not engaging their attention. Sometimes BPD people might even seem like they are "picking a fight" just to liven things up. If they win, they do not understand why the loser feels bad, but feel extremely hurt and betrayed if someone else wins instead.

These individuals have little skill at honest self-reflection. They do not have a realistic sense of their strengths and weaknesses, and will blame others rather than consider that they themselves have contributed to the situation. When you first meet someone with BPD, you might wonder why she does not have more friends, or a better career—yet after a time, you might feel that you understand why.

There can be a vicious cycle, in that those with BPD tend to turn others off—or else *get* turned off to others—and so, feeling abandoned, they think that nobody likes them. And so they do not get support that might help them to break the cycle.

Connection to Bipolar Disorder

Not only can BPD afflict the bipolar person, but its symptoms can sometimes be misconstrued as indications of bipolar disorder. Though the episodes are shorter and less intense, they involve many familiar elements of mania—such as sudden mood swings over seemingly nothing, risky spending and sex, and extreme impatience. The fundamental unhappiness and possible suicide attempts signal a similarity with some of the symptoms of depression.

 Fact

Dialectical behavior therapy (DBT) is a common method for treating BPD. A goal is to get patients to view the things they say and do— and the things that subsequently happen to them—in less extreme terms, and embrace more of a middle ground in life. Antidepressants and mood stabilizers are also sometimes used, in concert with individual and group therapy.

If a bipolar person also has BPD, they might be especially vulnerable to making sudden changes that the bipolar person is often wise to *not* make. For example, a rude nurse might seem like a valid reason to discontinue medication for an individual with BPD (though of course it is not).

Attention Deficit Hyperactivity Disorder (AD/HD)

AD/HD has been extensively researched and diagnosed in regard to children. Such youngsters find it difficult to sit still or concentrate, and thus often have problems in school. Medications such as Ritalin are commonly prescribed, though there is a minority opinion that such powerful medication should not be given to children, and that they should instead be trained in how to reorganize their thoughts. But what has received less attention is the reality of AD/HD in adults.

Less Obvious with Maturity

The adult with AD/HD does not necessarily squirm around like a child; many people simply become more composed as adults, at least on the surface. So sometimes it is mistakenly assumed that a child has "outgrown" the disorder. However, the symptoms become more internalized with age; hyperactive children often grow into more seemingly relaxed adults. Thus, it is often less obvious that an adult is experiencing AD/HD.

Essential

Adults with AD/HD are sometimes prescribed medication. But they also are often encouraged to pick careers that involve a minimum of repetition. They also are advised to exercise during breaks to work off excess energy, and make use of technology as needed. For example, if you think your mind will wander during an important lecture, use a tape recorder.

Moreover, there are of course children who are never diagnosed, so as adults they may not even know that it has ever been a problem with them. Instead, these people might spend a lifetime wondering why they never seem to be able to hold on to what they have.

Problems with Repetition

AD/HD is somewhat like having some of the symptoms of BPD. For example, boredom over repetition is common. This can be an issue in various areas of life:

- **Work:** People with AD/HD are likely to switch jobs often—or even get fired. If even the most interesting of jobs occasionally involves drudgery, these people are likely to overreact to how torturous it seems. When possible, they will probably try to get out of doing anything that sounds tedious; if they do show up, it will be hard to keep them focused on the task.
- **Romantic relationships:** Anything that gets too steady and predictable can seem "boring." AD/HD people might intentionally

wreck a relationship with infidelity or cruel complaints, just to feel free of the repetition of it.

- **Money:** Long-term planning does not interest people with AD/HD, and technical business language causes them to tune out. Even just balancing the checkbook can be a major chore. They might believe they are more or less keeping track of how much money they have, but then forget they wrote some other check.

- **Basic responsibilities:** Having to go to the grocery store and pick up clothes at the cleaners on the same day can seem overwhelming. Procrastination is preferred to facing a complex task that feels overwhelming. Even simpler things like picking clothes up off the floor or writing a letter can try their attention span.

One difference between AD/HD and BPD is that people with AD/HD do not make the same kinds of quick, negative value judgments against others. What is likelier is that they get angry from their general state of restlessness. Indeed, many AD/HD people are quick to anger. But since they cannot stay focused for long, they are equally quick to get over their anger. But other AD/HD people can actually seem more relaxed than the general population, depending on their circumstances. If things are going "well," they might be hyper with a kind of rapture. In any case, others might marvel at how rapidly these people can go from annoyed to content—and back again. Often, such people upset others without understanding why, since they themselves have long since forgotten whatever it was about.

Connection to Bipolar Disorder

The symptoms of adults with AD/HD might seem to resemble some of the manic or hypomanic tendencies. These would include being unable to concentrate for long, impatiently interrupting others, mismanagement of money, sudden bursts of anger, and making many sudden changes and decisions in one's personal or professional life.

Also, the frustration experienced over trying to get organized or finish things might at times seem like a lapse into depression and despair.

Question

What basic things can a person with AD/HD do to improve her situation?
Adults with AD/HD are encouraged to seek help from loved ones in organizing activities. Other helpful suggestions include: set obtainable goals and meet them; use calendars, daily lists, and other organizing tools; and strive to finish one goal before starting on another one.

A bipolar person who also has AD/HD will need to work extra hard at staying focused. Medications such as Ritalin can heighten mania, and so should be used extremely cautiously, if at all.

Post-Traumatic Stress Disorder (PTSD)

PTSD emerges after an exceptionally traumatizing event. These events can include being raped, tortured, or seriously injured; being kidnapped or abducted; watching someone get murdered; witnessing or experiencing a serious accident or bombing; getting caught in a natural disaster that causes great damage; and child abuse.

Dealing with Trauma

Many people are forced to experience horrific events. However sometimes, in the moment, people put some of their reaction on hold—they do not face the full reality of it. Perhaps the event is simply too large to fully comprehend all at once. Or maybe to survive, they must draw upon a deep inner courage and somehow get past the horror of the moment. In any case, it is as though they never finished processing what happened, and so they keep reliving it. There are several basic possibilities here.

With the right therapy and support network, some people might reach a point where the past rarely troubles them. However, sometimes the past event simply looms too large to ever fully recover from it. But some people learn to accept this. They know that what happened was not their own fault, and may even think that there would be something wrong if they *could* forget it all. Often, engaging in some sort of constructive social action to prevent whatever happened to them from happening to someone else proves helpful here.

Other people never do make any sort of peace with the past event. Sometimes they try but are unable to, and in other instances they might be in denial that anything bothers them—or that anything bad even happened. Such people might be unable to work, maintain relationships, or function very well in society. These are the people for whom PTSD is a long-term, even dangerous proposition.

Reminders of the Past

People with PTSD are extremely frightened by anything that reminds them of the traumatic incident, and will often avoid anything that does. Anniversaries of the past event might be especially traumatic. Someone who mysteriously bows out of an activity at the last moment when it seems to make no sense at all to do so might secretly be experiencing PTSD.

The trigger into the past horror can be something so small that it might not even be consciously remembered. For example, if as a child you were kidnapped and while being abducted there was a jingle on the radio for a certain brand of chewing gum, years later you might be upset when you see an ad for that brand of chewing gum, without understanding why.

Sometimes, though, the trigger is more obvious—for example, the sound of a gunshot. Given the tolerance for violence in our present culture, it can be difficult to avoid these kinds of reminders. Sometimes people who scrupulously avoid violence on TV or in movies are not just being "politically correct." Instead, they might *literally* be unable to stand watching anything that reminds them of being raped or molested, or seeing someone get shot to death, or whatever tragedy occurred to traumatize them.

Alert

People who are very sensitive—who feel more than others through the five senses—are more likely to experience PTSD. There will be that many more words, visual images, sounds, tastes, smells, sensations, and voices that conjure up the past.

When the trauma surfaces, the symptoms include flashbacks, in which they re-experience the trauma, often with sounds and visions. Anxiety and depression are also common. These episodes often last a month or more.

People with PTSD are often too frightened or embarrassed to explain what is going on, or why. Even when loved ones know what they went through, the afflicted people might think they are being a burden by bothering others with "all that" again. And so social relationships often become strained. Not surprisingly, people often turn to substance abuse to counter these feelings, and so addiction is common.

Connection to Bipolar Disorder

The sights, sounds, smells, touches, and tastes that trigger an episode of PTSD might seem perfectly normal and harmless to the non-sufferer. Thus, the suddenness of the depression or anxiety that comes with PTSD—perhaps even with hallucinatory flashbacks— might seem similar to someone undergoing an attack of bipolar depression. Substance abuse can also mimic or exacerbate both mania and depression.

If someone is bipolar and also has PTSD, she should make sure her psychiatrist is aware of the tragic events from her past, and whether or not she sometimes relives these events. That way, PTSD can be sorted out from bipolar disorder in determining what treatment is or is not working.

Ⱡ.. Essential

People from all walks of life can experience PTSD. But looking at the symptoms, it is not surprising that war veterans are especially vulnerable. Veterans of the Vietnam War are upward of fifty times more likely than other U.S. men to be homeless, to suffer from mood disorders, to be unable to work, and to have attempted suicide.

Intermittent Explosive Disorder (IED)

Everyone loses his temper sometimes; but IED episodes are intense and sudden attacks of anger and rage that go beyond what would seem to be a normal response to the situation at hand. The person with IED is not always full of rage, and sometimes responds with an appropriate degree of displeasure. But then come violent outbursts in which the individual loses all control of his aggressive impulses. Such people can cause serious damage to person or property. It has been suggested that many instances of assault or murder stem from IED. Some sources see it as a contributing factor in the recent outbreak of high school shootings.

Episodes begin and end quite abruptly. They can last for minutes or for hours. Commonly, people break objects or destroy property; they can also injure themselves or others. During an episode of IED, an individual often feels extremely confused, as though confusion were fueling the rage. Such people may even later report amnesia-like symptoms, and not remember what they just did.

Typically, people are contrite and apologetic once the episode is over. They may remorsefully promise to never do it again—but these promises are rarely kept.

Diagnosing IED

IED is a kind of default diagnosis. That is to say, the diagnosis is made when it is apparent that no other disorder is a better explanation. The person absolutely does not have other kinds of symptoms associated with other kinds of disorders. It also is apparent that the symptoms cannot be blamed on alcohol or drug abuse. In other words, the afflicted individual might otherwise seem "normal" but for these extremely troubling outbursts of temper. This might make it difficult to ever get diagnosed, because both the individual and others might instead keep hoping that it simply never happens again.

Once diagnosed, IED might be treated by medication, therapy, or both. There is some evidence to suggest it is neurological in nature. It is not uncommon to see abnormal EEGs in these patients.

Connection to Bipolar Disorder

People in a manic or depressive phase might display sudden rage over seemingly nothing. If deluded or hallucinating, they might well be confused, and afterward remember at best only some of what they did. The remorse experienced after an IED episode might be confused with depression. Thus, it is important that a thorough evaluation be made as to what is or is not happening, so that someone who is bipolar not be misdiagnosed IED—or vice versa.

 ## Alert

One of the more common manifestations of IED is "road rage." Drivers go out of their way to hit other vehicles or drive them off the road, sometimes resulting in serious injury or death. The behavior of the other driver is really just a catalyst for anger over some deeper issue. Males in their thirties are the likeliest perpetrators of road rage.

Seasonal Affective Disorder (SAD)

SAD is depression caused by seasonal change. Specifically, some people become depressed during the winter months, when there is relatively little sunlight.

SAD seems to be related to one's natural circadian (or daily) rhythm. These rhythms change with the seasons, but for some people the changes in the winter seem out of sync. A sleep hormone called melatonin is also associated with depression. Melatonin is more rapidly produced in the dark, and so individuals might produce more melatonin during the winter—and for some people, "too much" is produced.

Peak winter months are the most difficult, but SAD symptoms can start up as early as the fall. The condition lessens come the spring, and over the summer months is gone. (There sometimes are hypomanic-like symptoms in the first four weeks of spring.)

Thus, to be diagnosed as having SAD, most or all of one's depression must be experienced during the winter months, and there should be virtually never any depression over the summer months. People who live close to the equator would not experience SAD, because there are long, sunny days year round.

Symptoms of SAD

People with SAD often have an increased need for sleep. Sometimes, too, sleep is disturbed by unhappily awakening in the early morning. The reasons might be bad dreams or a general anxiousness. And like other expressions of depression, SAD people feel hopeless, guilty, and unworthy. There is an intense lethargy, and a lack of desire to carry out daily tasks. Stressful situations seem impossible to confront. Sexual desire diminishes. SAD people also have exceptionally large appetites for sugars and starches; excessive winter weight gain is not uncommon. The immune system seems weakened, and people are especially vulnerable to infection and disease.

Connection to Bipolar Disorder

Obviously, both SAD and bipolar disorder involve depression, and the symptoms of depression, per se, can be similar. Additionally, the rather hypomanic conditions come the spring suggest a further parallel with bipolar disorder. Bipolar people sensitive to changes in seasons should make their doctor aware of this.

 ## Fact

> Bright-light therapy, or phototherapy, is usually used to treat SAD. Commonly, this treatment involves a row of fluorescent lights attached to a metal reflector. Also, some research has shown that an hour of walking in the sunshine during winter works as well as over two hours under the fluorescent lights. In either case, the goal is to lessen melatonin secretions in the brain.

Looking at SAD and other mood disorders, it is not difficult to see how other disorders can be both similar to and different from bipolar. It also is not hard to see how the existence of these various disorders can complicate diagnosis and treatment. However, a psychiatrist is trained to sort these disorders out, and see which one(s), if any, apply to you. As with other forms of depression, treatment can inadvertently produce mania or hypomania. With good doctor-patient interaction, the right diagnosis and treatment can be found.

CHAPTER 4

Who Gets Bipolar Disorder?

Not everyone is equally vulnerable to bipolar disorder. Physical factors, such as gender, ethnicity, and age, are thought to influence a person's tendency toward bipolar disorder. There is also a question as to whether or not being bipolar is related to creativity. Those who believe so wonder whether or not treatment for bipolar disorder therefore limits creativity. This chapter will cover all the different facts and figures surrounding who gets the disorder.

Important Factors

It is not known exactly how many people in the United States are bipolar, since many people never see a psychiatrist and remain undiagnosed. But as mentioned earlier, bipolar disorder seems to be present in about 1 to 5 percent of the total population—at the very least, 2 million people. Following are some more demographics.

Gender

Bipolar disorder affects both women and men, but there are some slight differences in the way each gender manifests and handles it. Women are more likely to first seek treatment for depression, while men are more likely to seek treatment for mania. Men seem to be slightly more likely to experience both Bipolar I and II over the course of a lifetime—about 4 percent of men become bipolar versus about 3 percent of women (though, again, these figures might be slightly conservative). Evidence also suggests that men are more likely than women to have Bipolar I than II by a rate of about two to one.

Fact

Contrary to a popular rumor, the Amish are no more likely to be bipolar than any other group. However, the Amish have been used in studies of bipolar disorder because of their detailed records of lineage that go back for centuries. This makes it easier to study the genetic components of bipolar disorder, as well as track bipolar symptoms in children.

Bipolar women are possibly more likely to have developed alcohol dependency and to attempt suicide. At the same time, bipolar men are slightly more likely to have had a history of violence and legal problems. But of course, both men and women can and do experience all of these conditions.

Ethnicity and Age

Ethnically speaking, Native Americans appear to be the likeliest group to acquire bipolar disorder—the rate is about 8 percent. Next come African Americans (slightly over 4 percent), Asian/Pacific Islanders (4 percent), with Hispanic Americans and European Americans both at slightly over 3 percent.

Age-wise, young adults (aged eighteen to twenty-four) have the highest reported rates of bipolar disorder, approaching 10 percent. The known rate decreases to between 4 and 3 percent for adults aged twenty-five to forty-four. It then varies between 2 and 1 percent for people forty-five to sixty-four. The rate further decreases to a mere half of a percent for people sixty-five or older. We can only speculate whether more young people are being sent to doctors, or whether the actual rate of the illness is somehow increasing. (Since substance abuse and other social factors can hasten the presence of bipolar disorder, the latter should not be discounted as a possibility.)

In any case, bipolar disorder tends to first strike in someone's teens or early twenties—though some recent evidence suggests that more people are affected by it during childhood than was thought. Depressed children might be more likely to become bipolar adults.

Geography and Economics

In the United States, the Southeast sees the highest incidence of bipolar disorder—a solid 5 percent. New Englanders see the least bipolar—just over 2 percent. Contrary to what might be expected, larger cities have lower rates of bipolar disorder than medium-sized ones. Cities with populations between 100,000 and 500,000 have a rate of over 4 percent—as do rural areas—while cities with more than 2 million only have a rate of over 2 percent.

There are economic patterns as well. Households with incomes of less than $20,000 have a rate of almost 6 percent. By contrast, households of $85,000 or more have a rate of less than 2 percent. The size of the household is also revealing. Households of one have a rate of over 2 percent, while households of five or more have a rate of nearly 5 percent. While lifestyle does not cause bipolar disorder, it can serve to increase or decrease the likelihood or intensity of its presence. Perhaps lower-income people—and larger families—face more daily life stressors, and therefore have a higher rate of bipolar disorder.

About 50 percent of all bipolar people attempt suicide, and about 85 percent will be hospitalized for bipolar disorder at least once.

Are Some People More Likely to Be Bipolar?

There is increasing evidence that bipolar disorder is genetic in origin. If someone in your family is bipolar, there is greater chance that someone else will be, too.

The good news is that we know more than ever about the genetic component in bipolar disorder. Immediate family members (parents and siblings) of a bipolar person are more likely to also be bipolar than persons from families without an immediate bipolar family member. And people with a bipolar relative from a previous generation are more likely to be bipolar than people who do not have such a relative. All told, people with either a diagnosed bipolar relative or at least a family history of mood instability account for over 90 percent of the diagnosed bipolar cases.

The bad news is two-fold. First, many people are undoubtedly concerned to hear that bipolar disorder can run in families. Also, however, this information does not always tell the average person as much as it should. Many people do not know their genetic lineage very far back.

Furthermore, there are those who come from families in which no one was ever diagnosed because people did not often go to doctors—and *never* to psychiatrists. Many people can only speculate whether that high-strung relative who sometimes turned violent had undiagnosed bipolar disorder—or if it was some other problem. So, relatively few people can say with absolute certainty that they are or are not genetically predisposed to bipolar disorder.

 Alert

Manic children are more likely to be angry and destructive than euphoric. Depressive children often complain of aches and tiredness, whine a great deal, fear rejection, and at least talk about running away from home—and often do. These children also are likely to engage in alcohol and drug abuse.

In any case, it would seem that some people *are* genetically predisposed to bipolar disorder. It also appears to be true that different kinds of upheavals and lifestyle issues can make bipolar more or less likely to manifest in such an individual. We will be discussing these factors in more detail in future chapters. But for now, be aware that substance abuse, unsettling childhoods, major changes and upheavals, and diet can all make a difference. Bipolar symptoms are also found in over 50 percent of the cases of postpartum depression.

To use an example: If, tragically, you were sexually abused as a child but survived your twenties *without* experiencing truly dramatic mood swings, there is a good chance that you will *not* have to worry about being bipolar. The rage expressed by your abusive father was possibly not bipolar disorder but something else, such as alcoholism.

Famous Bipolar People

In recent decades, a range of well-known people have become known as bipolar. This is often publicized to help educate the public, or to show that bipolar disorder does not have to stop you from achieving success in life. In other instances, the information comes to light through second-hand sources, or even after the person has died—sometimes having committed suicide.

A wide range of actors has been associated with bipolar disorder, including Ned Beatty, Patty Duke, Carrie Fisher, Linda Hamilton, Mariette Hartley, Margot Kidder, Vivien Leigh, Kevin McDonald, Kristy McNichol, Michael Moriarity, Jason Robards, Rod Steiger, Ben Stiller, and Jean-Claude Van Damme. There have also been distinguished directors said to be bipolar, including Tim Burton, Francis Ford Coppola, and Joshua Logan. (Duke, Robards, Steiger, and Coppola have all won Academy Awards.)

From the world of music, persons alleged to be bipolar include pop singers Rosemary Clooney and Connie Francis, country star Charley Pride, and rock musicians Kurt Cobain, Ray Davies, Axl Rose, Sting, and Brian Wilson.

Still other well-known personalities that have been considered bipolar include astronaut Buzz Aldrin, humorist Art Buchwald, television personality Dick Cavett, controversial magazine publisher Larry Flynt, left-wing activist Abbie Hoffman, musician-raconteur Oscar Levant, and news host Jane Pauley.

Much has been speculated about famous people of the past who might have suffered from bipolar disorder. So much more is known now about mental illness that information about who was considered "sick" or "normal" in the past must be taken with a proverbial grain of salt. Relatively little was known about mental illness, including how to diagnose it or treat it. Sometimes, people were diagnosed mentally ill when it was really just that they were victims of highly conservative values that did not permit them to be themselves. Likewise, there had to have been many people who because of their name, privilege, or ability to conform were never diagnosed as mentally ill when they should have been.

 Fact

The guessing game of bipolar versus other disorders is reflected in two legends: Marilyn Monroe and Judy Garland. Biographies on these famous stars make note of eating and sleeping problems, as well dramatic mood swings. Yet both stars also had issues with alcohol and drugs. So was it bipolar disorder made more pronounced by substance abuse, or just substance abuse?

Nonetheless, there is quite a list of artists, writers, and musicians who apparently suffered at least from some form of unipolar depression, and who also may have been bipolar.

From the world of art, Michelangelo, Paul Gauguin, Vincent van Gogh, Georgia O'Keeffe, Jackson Pollock, and Mark Rothko are all on the list. Poets include Charles Baudelaire, John Berryman, William Blake, Robert Burns, George Gordon, Lord Byron, Hart Crane, Emily Dickinson, T. S. Eliot, Vachel Lindsay, Robert Lowell, Sylvia Plath, Edgar Allan Poe, Ezra Pound, Anne Sexton, Percy Bysshe Shelley, Alfred Lord Tennyson, Dylan Thomas, and Walt Whitman. Novelists such as Samuel Clemens (Mark Twain), Joseph Conrad, Charles Dickens, Isak Dinesen, William Faulkner, F. Scott Fitzgerald, Graham Greene, Ernest Hemingway, Victor Hugo, Henry James, Herman Melville, Boris Pasternak, Mary Shelley, Robert Louis Stevenson, Leo Tolstoy, Virginia Woolf, and Emile Zola are also frequently mentioned.

Also included on the list are playwrights Noel Coward, Henrik Ibsen, William Inge, Eugene O'Neill, and Tennessee Williams; along with children's authors Hans Christian Andersen and James M. Barrie; philosopher Ralph Waldo Emerson; composers Irving Berlin and Cole Porter; and jazz legends Charles Mingus and Charles Parker.

Bipolar and Creativity

The highly impressive list of names that might be associated with bipolar disorder begs the question, Is bipolar somehow connected to being talented and creative? For centuries people have wondered if talent or genius are somehow linked to "madness." Gifted people often seem more sensitive or high-strung, and often report feeling somehow "different." More to the point, many creative people have a history of being under a doctor's care, or commitment to a mental hospital (often following a suicide attempt). Some are even diagnosed bipolar.

In actuality, the percentage of highly creative people who probably have bipolar disorder is something like 40 percent, or about ten times higher than the general population. Obviously, there are many bipolar people who are *not* famous artists, or even particularly talented in the arts. But if someone is artistically renowned, she is more likely to be bipolar (or have another mental disorder) than someone who is not.

How Creativity Manifests in Bipolar People

Bipolar disorder takes people on a journey to the highest of highs and the lowest of lows. This can wreak havoc upon the self and others. But if someone can use these experiences artistically, she is able to express deep feeling and insight into the human experience. If it is true that in order to move an audience an artist must have suffered, bipolar disorder ironically can provide a treasure of creativity. Certainly bipolar people should be encouraged to use their experiences in ways that can move or inspire others.

But the creativity comes at a high price—the suicide rate among artists is likewise about ten times as high as in the general population, with bipolar disorder being a prime cause of these untimely deaths. And suicide is the obvious opposite of creativity.

Essential

In many ways, the question of bipolar's connection to creativity remains a riddle of the chicken or the egg: Would a given individual have been an actor, painter, or writer anyway, or did his experiences with bipolar disorder move him in that direction?

Does Treatment Destroy Creativity?

While some people worry that going on medication will turn them into "zombies" or "vegetables," those who make their living being creative generally report that this is not true.

Popular treatments for bipolar disorder such as lithium (which will be discussed in Chapter 6) sometimes result in a certain diminishing of the senses—what has been described as a "flattening out" of life. But almost 60 percent of the artistic people on lithium and other drugs report their creativity actually *increased* once medicated—and another 20 percent report that it stayed about the same.

Slightly over 20 percent do report a decrease in creativity. It is extremely difficult to know how another person experiences life. But perhaps sometimes this "flattening out" is really just a matter of eliminating the heightened, exaggerated perceptions that often accompany bipolar disorder. One person's "flat" might be someone else's "normal."

More importantly, if people need not experience long periods of being unable to function—let alone that they no longer attempt suicide—they indeed might increase their creative output over time. A life lived relatively normally will still have to withstand many a crisis; one certainly need not have a bipolar episode in order to learn from life.

Of this 20 percent who report diminished creativity, it is possible that some might be trying to fight treatment. But even if none of them are, perhaps the best that can be said is that while treatment has come a long way, it is still being refined and improved upon. Hopefully, future medications will not have this effect at all.

Fact

Besides people in the arts, famous statesmen have also been studied for evidence of unipolar or bipolar symptoms. Abraham Lincoln, Theodore Roosevelt, and Winston Churchill are among the colorful and important men of history who had documented instances of dramatic shifts of mood that required the care of a doctor.

Can Bipolar People Have a Normal Life?

With so many famous people associated with bipolar disorder, it might seem as though it enables people to succeed in their goals. But this is hardly the case. About a third to a half of the people with bipolar disorder do not work, and just as many are supported through social services. Still, there are things you can do to ensure a more normal life with bipolar disorder.

A Look at the Past and Present

Present-day people who are famous and successful do not escape the basic reality of either finding the right treatment and having to stick to it, or else experiencing episodes of extreme embarrassment, pain, and danger because they are not being treated. And fame and fortune have never prevented anyone from committing suicide. It may well be (as was discussed in Chapter 2) that our contemporary world applauds overachievement. But people still must learn to live with themselves once the applause fades away.

As for famous people in the past who seemed to "get away with" being bipolar, it cannot be underemphasized that many of them were frequently hospitalized for their profound unhappiness—and many even took their own lives.

Moreover, there is a different social world now—one that makes it evermore difficult to succeed at anything without good "people skills." In the communication era, it becomes increasingly more important to be able to communicate well with an ever-wider range of people. While society becomes increasingly informed and tolerant of mental conditions, it also continually raises the bar of expectation regarding the people affected by them.

This is true not only in the professional world, but the personal as well. People live longer than ever before. Most people marry out of love and personal choice instead of having marriages arranged by families. There are high expectations for the quality of life. What all this means is that if someone does not get along with their co-workers or clients, they are likely to get fired. When people no longer love their spouses, they get divorced. Someone with a bad temper might be ordered to take anger management classes, or see a therapist.

 Alert

Frequently, bipolar children are misdiagnosed as having AD/HD. What makes this especially unfortunate is that the medications often prescribed for this are stimulants that exacerbate the bipolar symptoms. It is also possible for a child to be both bipolar and to have AD/HD.

A hundred years ago, people did not live as long, there was much less knowledge about mental disorders, and divorce was much more frowned upon. If a man had a bad temper but was a good baker (for example), the family figured, "Oh well, he sells his bread and supports us." And customers might have said, "He's rude, but his bread tastes good." In today's world, it is less likely that people would feel obligated to tolerate this behavior.

It is also true that creative people of a past era came from wealthy families, or had benefactors. Many, again, also did not live very long, and so did not have to worry about how to support themselves over a lifetime.

Thus, finding treatment in today's world for bipolar is even more important than ever. But here is where it gets complicated: It would be wonderful it if could be reported that everyone diagnosed bipolar finds the right combination of medication, and goes on to live a life free of future episodes. But such is not the case.

The Question of Treatment

At a basic level, a distinction can be made between bipolar people who get treatment and bipolar people who do not. Those who do not even try a treatment regime are absolutely setting themselves up for future episodes.

As for those who do seek treatment, data on success rates can vary. Even older medications get re-tested constantly, let alone newer ones. There also is the matter of multiple medications to treat multiple symptoms, and this further complicates both treatment and research.

You will learn more about issues that emerge around treatment in more detail in subsequent chapters. But for now, it could be said that upward of 60 percent of the patients medicated for bipolar disorder respond favorably to treatment.

However, there is no guarantee that they will remain absolutely symptom-free, or that adjustments or new combinations of medication will not be needed. Over 10 percent of bipolar patients who initially respond to a given medication will fail to do so over time. Something like 30 percent of the patients report negative side effects from one or more medications. Regular check-ups with a psychiatrist are essential.

On balance, medication is not a cure-all, but the difference between medication and no medication can literally be a matter of life and death. Even partial freedom from bipolar symptoms should not be lightly dismissed. With a strong support system, an honest relationship with a doctor, and a willingness to try, the majority of bipolar people are able to accomplish much more than they might have thought.

Essential

Some research indicates that the average patient is now prescribed three medications at a time. The effectiveness of a given medication therefore becomes not just how it treats symptoms per se, but how well it does or does not interact with other medications prescribed.

Putting Bipolar into Perspective

It is perfectly natural for people to try to understand why things happen in their lives. Since the dawn of humanity, explanations have been offered as to why there is human suffering. However, a down side of this type of thinking is that it assumes that (a) there is only one reason for why anything happens, and (b) we are fully capable of knowing what this reason is.

The genetic basis of bipolar disorder, in and of itself provides a powerful explanation as to "why" someone is bipolar: it is in her DNA. No deity, force, or person was somehow trying to punish her.

Remember: Everyone develops maladies, ailments, or problematic habits over a life course. As the old saying goes, no one gets a free ride. Living with bipolar is not always easy, and frequently it is difficult. Yet the same could be said for any other serious mental or physical issue—as well as life tragedies, such as the premature death of a loved one. If you are bipolar, by all means treat it with the utmost seriousness. But also remember that other people have their own burdens to bear.

Also, if you respond well to treatment, you have less to complain about than many a lost soul. Since bipolar *is* now treatable in the majority of cases, one might at least appreciate not being bipolar, say, a hundred years ago. And remember, too, that many other ailments are not yet treatable at all.

Ideally, medications that eliminate bipolar symptoms in all patients—and with a minimum of side effects—will be developed. Perhaps as our understanding of the causes of bipolar disorder continues to grow, there will even be a cure. But in the meantime, there is solace in the progress that has been made.

CHAPTER 5

What Causes Bipolar Disorder?

Learning what causes an illness does much more than satisfy intellectual curiosity. It can also aid in finding treatment, or even an eventual cure. Great strides have been made in uncovering the roots of bipolar disorder—how and why it manifests in certain people. These causes would seem to be largely biological in nature, though social forces and experiences also play a role. In years to come, doubtless even more will be known about the factors that make people bipolar.

Nature Versus Nurture: The Endless Debate

Virtually any illness is subject to the ongoing debate of nature versus nurture—or heredity versus environment. In particular, mental disorders might be debated, since indeed one person's rage (for example) might be a matter of social experiences, while another's is a matter of brain chemicals—or perhaps a combination of both.

Contrasting Beliefs

A TV news show might one moment have a segment on chemical breakthrough in cancer research—and the next moment another segment on how attitude can aid in the healing process. Anytime someone claims there is a biological explanation for something, there is another person ready to counter that the problem at hand is purely psychological. Seen in this light, it makes perfect sense that despite increasing evidence that bipolar disorder has a genetic basis, there are those who remain unconvinced. This disbelief takes several forms.

At a basic level, there are those who believe that virtually nothing should be treated chemically. Instead, they feel that there should always be some sort of natural remedy—be it diet, exercise, a belief system, an engaging hobby, or talking therapy. (In fact, all of these might well help the bipolar person, and should not be discounted—but neither should drug treatment.)

Similarly, there are those who do not trust psychiatry. Some people think that bipolar disorder is just something that doctors invented to take patients' money. Or they think that some people enjoy having a fancy mental diagnosis because it gets them more attention, or gives them license to make excuses for themselves. Still other people cannot get beyond their own life experience. Since *they* have never lost total control of their emotions, no one else should have to do so. And if they themselves have been through some rough times, they might be that much less sympathetic. Such people think: "If anyone knows what it's like to have high highs and low lows, it's me—but you just have to get over it."

Essential

Disbelief also emerges from actual experiences with the medical community. Sometimes a doctor will re-test someone for bipolar disorder, and conclude that the person is not bipolar after all. Or one doctor might say the person is, and then a second doctor might think the problem is something else. The effect of this can be that the patient concludes that since he himself was not really bipolar, probably anyone who is diagnosed bipolar is not really bipolar, either.

Additionally, people sometimes engage in the all-too-familiar phenomenon of denial. Some people have extreme difficulty admitting there is anything wrong with anyone—even a total stranger on a TV talk show. Sometimes there simply is a reluctance to embrace the more challenging aspects of life; people find it "upsetting" to ponder that there are those who actually have serious problems. But in other instances, people have a great deal of internalized shame over illness—especially mental illness—and consider it a sign of weakness.

Disbelief Perpetuates the Problem

With all due respect for difference of opinion, stubborn disbelief often results in perpetuating shame and misunderstanding about what bipolar disorder actually is—or is not. Bipolar disorder is *not* simply a matter of being confused, intense, or neurotic. The data on the harsh realities of bipolar signal that sole reliance on nonmedication is dangerously naïve.

At the same time, you can be someone who *tends to* have strong feelings, or *tends to* feel either optimistic or pessimistic, without being bipolar. Instead, you might simply be quite sensitive to changes in your everyday life. If you feel insecure as to how much other people like you, your problem might have more to do with social skills or past events. Once again, this in itself does not make you bipolar.

People who get treated for bipolar disorder and later talk about it often emphasize that it is difficult to articulate just what the cycle feels like—other than to say that it does *not* feel like normal, everyday changes of mood. The manic swings are *not* the same thing as drinking too many cups of coffee; the depressive part of the cycle is *not* the same thing as needing a little cheering up.

 Fact

A model employed to describe this interplay of heredity and environment is the Diathesis-Stress Model. "Diathesis" refers to a physical predisposition toward a certain symptom or disease. The "stress" factor here refers to stressors from the environment. When someone has a genetic predisposition to bipolar disorder but does not develop the symptoms, it is called incomplete penetrance.

What further complicates the issue is the fact that the genetic evidence is still a work in progress. For example, studies on bipolar in identical twins have revealed that both members of the set do not always develop bipolar symptoms. The rate of both being bipolar is quite high, perhaps even 80 percent. But it is *not* at 100 percent; other factors play a role.

On balance, life events interface with genetic predisposition in the formation of a bipolar individual. As in other areas of life, *both* nature and nurture are important.

Genetics and Bipolar Disorder

Recent research has concluded that there are specific genetic components involved in the transmission of bipolar disorder. And more is being learned all the time.

Chromosomes

Chromosomes are contained in cells within the DNA structure, and they carry the genes that determine one's sex and other characteristics. There are twenty-three pairs of chromosomes in a human being's DNA. The chromosomes that transmit what becomes bipolar disorder include the X chromosome, and chromosome eleven. While more is still being learned as to the nature and purpose of chromosomes, the X chromosome also carries hemophilia, and chromosome eleven apparently also carries sickle cell anemia.

The genetic coding that these (or possibly other) chromosomes carry in regard to bipolar disorder would seem to be related to how the brain receives certain messages. Through techniques such as magnetic resonance imaging (MRI), there is evidence that there are differences between the brains of bipolar people and non-bipolar people. For example, in bipolar people, there appear to be 30 percent more brain cells in certain areas of the brain that send messages to other areas of the brain. This might well account for the heightened sensations experienced when moods go up or down.

Neurotransmitters and Other Factors

Other research has focused on the actual chemicals that function as *neurotransmitters*, or the messengers within the brain. These neurotransmitters include serotonin, dopamine, and norepinephrine. Perhaps high or low levels of these substances cause the brain to get different images and information than "normal" people do. This may also involve the strength or weakness of one compound in relation to another.

Essential

While it is now well established that many illnesses are genetically transmitted, at one time the medical community thought otherwise. Prominent psychiatrists such as Karl Menninger (co-founder of the Menninger Clinic) strongly advocated that no attempts be made to classify mental illness—that it was all basically the same, and all required psychoanalysis, or talk therapy, to be treated.

Additional research has focused on possible change in nerve-cell receptors. These receptors possibly become more sensitive in bipolar people. And so a "whisper," so to speak, is received as a "shout."

Thus, just as being musically inclined might run in a family, so do certain illnesses and disorders. If you have the potential to be a good musician but never get a chance to play an instrument, the proclivity will remain dormant. Similarly, social conditions and behavior will inhibit or encourage the manifestation of bipolar disorder.

Physiology: How the Body Works

The brain is a body organ, so mental responses are also physical in nature. Therefore, the physiological interplay of pure biology and human perception and behavior is important in understanding the origins and nature of bipolar disorder.

Bipolar and Childbirth

Bipolar disorder appears to be related to several issues surrounding childbirth. Postpartum depression is an established scientific condition. However, research is finding that in upward of half the documented cases, the symptoms are not unipolar (solely depression) but bipolar (mania and depression). This signals that childbirth was the physiological trigger for these women, that they had an inherent tendency toward bipolar disorder, and having a child was the experience that brought forth an episode.

 Fact

Studies have revealed differences in the brains of bipolar persons. These differences involve the right, or non-dominant hemisphere of the brain, which is concerned with spatial and visual skills. Thus, bipolar people often score below average on tests of visual and spatial skills. Patients with schizophrenia are more likely to have impairments in the left hemisphere, which processes language.

Some recent studies have concluded that low birth weight is related to bipolar disorder. Whether the low birth weight is a cause or a symptom requires further research. However, prenatal famine has likewise been shown to be related to bipolar disorder. Obviously, low birth weight can result from prenatal famine, but other conditions can cause it as well. And not all low birth-rate babies develop bipolar disorder. More research is needed on these compelling issues.

Bipolar and Climate

There also is a growing body of evidence that climates with less sunshine not only increase the likelihood of SAD, but of bipolar episodes. In other words, living in a less sunny climate does not *cause* bipolar, but it might increase the number of episodes someone has.

The issue of climate and bipolar is a good example of how factors of nature versus nurture can be challenging to sort out. For example, many people tend to be more moody on non-sunny days, so perhaps for bipolar people this can mean taking things a step further into full-blown manic-depression. On the other hand, perhaps there are more complex bodily processes at work that have not yet been determined.

In any event, these and other studies point to the ways in which the essential genetic possibility of bipolar disorder might be more or less likely due to certain interplays of body and mind.

Life Experience Matters

A growing body of research indicates that particularly during childhood, body chemicals that affect the functioning of the brain or other vital organs can sometimes be altered in their intensity from certain traumatic events. Hence, the things that do or do not happen to people in their everyday lives can make it more or less likely that someone manifests bipolar disorder.

Abuse

Studies have shown that children and adolescents who are physically or sexually abused are more likely to manifest bipolar symptoms. Once again, the abuse does not *cause* bipolar disorder—if it did, many more people would be bipolar, because child abuse is sadly all too common in our society. Instead, there seem to be several plausible scenarios.

One possibility is that abuse brings bipolar tendencies to the surface. Some people might be born with a certain proclivity toward bipolar thinking and behavior. The trauma of the abuse might compel certain brain processes to realign themselves in ways that enable the inherent bipolar condition to emerge.

At the same time, bipolar children might be more likely to be abused. Impatient parents or guardians might lose their tempers with children whose destructive behavior seems totally unwarranted.

Thus, such children might receive excessive and unreasonable punishments. Also, a child might be sexually abused by a relative who takes advantage of the child's unstable nature and behavior.

Still another possible connection here is that children are likely to have poor coping skills. Adults who suffered serious abuse as children might in general have difficulty coping with certain situations. And so if there are bipolar tendencies in an adult survivor of abuse, certain situations might in fact serve to trigger an episode.

Social Support

Other research has noted that bipolar adults with less social support are likely to have more episodes. This also points to the importance of the environment—though once again, there are different possible reasons for this.

First, social support can mean positive thoughts. Bipolar or not, all people make cognitive evaluations of the things they experience—and their cognitions can be altered by input from other people. This is why it is possible to genuinely comfort another person; it is possible to internalize what is said, and replace a former, negative perception with a new, positive one. It goes without saying that some life events are easier to cognitively realign than others. Still, having people around to convince you that everything will be okay, or something was not really so bad, can make a difference.

On the other hand, *not* having a strong support network can only increase the likelihood of exaggerated perceptions.

 Alert

Though there is much evidence to suggest that stressors from daily life events can trigger serious bipolar episodes, some sources call these conclusions into question. For example, it is argued that people claim that daily life issues caused an episode after the fact—at which time some people might be looking for an excuse for their behavior.

Additionally, social support can mean more understanding. A bipolar person with trusted friends who understand quite a lot about bipolar disorder might be less likely to slip into an episode. Medication is still the most important thing, but feeling loved and cared about, and having people to talk things over with, can only help. Also, of course, these loved ones can remind someone to take medication, drive the person to the doctor, and so on.

On the other hand, *not* having a strong social support network can make it less likely that someone will get the help needed when a crisis is looming.

Diet and Drugs

A healthy diet does not mean that bipolar symptoms will never appear. If all it took to cure bipolar disorder was an extra teaspoon of wheat germ, it would have ceased to be a problem years ago. So-called vitamin therapy might work for some things, but alas, it simply does not make bipolar symptoms go away. However, there might well be valid issues concerning bipolar disorder and diet—as well as drugs.

Essential

There is a popular misconception that eating too much sugar can cause diabetes. This is not true. However, too much sugar can cause obesity—and obesity is one of the factors that can contribute to Type II diabetes. Obesity is of course also associated with cardiovascular problems, and sets in motion other forms of physical ailments. It furthermore can negatively impact one's self-image—which again can trigger a host of other undesirable thoughts and behaviors.

Diet

A junk-food diet does not cause bipolar disorder. Still, a poor diet can make you more vulnerable to any number of ailments—which can mean more likelihood of unpleasant feelings and sensations, not to mention having to take medications that might interfere with bipolar treatment. While a bipolar episode can emerge over seemingly nothing, it is tempting fate to not pay attention to diet and nutrition if you are bipolar.

Blood sugar has been shown to effect mood. The high concentration of sugar in most junk foods can cause the average person's moods to go from high to low and back again. For the bipolar person, consuming vast quantities of junk food can be like playing with fire.

Drugs

It has been discussed elsewhere that so-called recreational drug use can often trigger the active presence of bipolar disorder. This can happen in several ways.

In the present moment, a recreational drug experience can trigger physiological responses that in turn make it more likely to experience a bipolar episode. Also, over time, drug use can have a collective effect of making someone with a tendency toward bipolar disorder experience more outright episodes.

Furthermore, altered mental states distort perceptions. High highs, low lows, and distorted perceptions are likely to occur when taking recreational drugs. Such states of being can only exacerbate the possibility of bipolar disorder.

When bipolar persons are prescribed drugs for other conditions, they should make certain that their physician knows the medications they take for bipolar, and learn about any possible drug interactions.

When the Unexpected Happens

Getting the proverbial rug pulled out from under your feet is never fun for anyone, but for the bipolar person it might trigger an episode. Sometimes an unexpected life event might even be part of what makes the disorder first manifest itself.

Rapid Changes

Dramatic or unexpected changes obviously affect everyone, whether the change be in one's personal or professional life. But these changes can have special meanings for bipolar people. For example, anyone would be devastated to suddenly be dropped by a significant other. Even people who normally behave quite reasonably might drink too much, be short-tempered or despondent. But for the bipolar person, these seemingly "normal" responses to losing a relationship can mean setting in motion an episode of mania or depression. Why this might cause depression seems obvious enough; it hurts to be rejected. But depression can lead to mania, whereby the person delves into grandiosity and the reckless behavior that accompanies it.

Even just dating someone new can sometimes dramatically dislocate the self. It can seem like a good thing, but it can also make for changes in one's routine and expose one to a challenging new set of expectations. The same can hold true for a new job, or a promotion.

Moving to a new community is almost always painful for children—but for a young person who is bipolar, it can be more than that. The fears that accompany normal social uncertainty can escalate to a more troubling level. And for adults, moving can mean keeping track of myriad plans. Counting boxes for movers while calling the utility company in another city can bring out the manic nature in *anyone*, let alone a bipolar person.

 Fact

Demographics show that people are likely to die within a year or two of retiring, often for no apparent reason other than an inability to adjust to the dramatic change of no longer going to work every day. For this reason, many companies have started to offer counseling services to employees who retire.

Furthermore, unfamiliar people might be less accustomed to knowing how to deal with the bipolar person—regardless of whether or not they know the person is bipolar, or the person has been having episodes. Thus, it is all the more likely that some new acquaintance will say or do something that the bipolar person does not know how to deal with.

Loss and Sorrow

Many people never get over the death of a loved one, the divorce of their parents—or their own divorce. Injuries, accidents, and illnesses that require long recuperation—or perhaps leave one permanently disabled—can likewise require intense mental and emotional adjustment. So when in addition to this traumatic experience itself, you are bipolar, the possibility for a major episode cannot be denied.

Once again, seemingly "normal" responses can have a special meaning for a bipolar person. Drinking, not eating or sleeping—or eating or sleeping too much—are behavioral patterns best avoided if you are bipolar. Tears of sorrow might lapse into depression. And if depression turns to mania, any number of unfortunate actions might be taken to deal with the loss at hand—spending binges, compulsive sex, or even murder.

Also, bipolar people need to be mindful of getting too involved in other people's issues. For example, in the immediate period following the demise of a relationship, most anyone can be quite tempted to obsess about what their ex-spouse is now thinking or doing. But for a bipolar person, this is a definite step in the wrong direction.

All people benefit from trying to keep their lives as organized and well-planned as possible. But it is also true that all people will still have to deal with the unexpected. For bipolar people, having a strong support network and a good relationship with a trained professional can prove especially useful when dealing with life's surprises.

CHAPTER 6

Treatment for Bipolar Disorder

Short of a cure, it would be wonderful if there were one medication that treated all of the bipolar symptoms for everyone—with virtually no side effects. But in the meantime, researchers try to find the best possible chemical compounds to treat as effectively as possible as many symptoms as possible—and with as few side effects as possible. These medications include mood stabilizers, antidepressants, antipsychotics, sleep aids, and anti-anxiety drugs. Often, patients are prescribed more than one medication.

History of Treatment

After the advent of Freud and the ongoing patient-doctor dialogues as therapy, some doctors thought that bipolar disorder could be talked through. In other words, it was a malady that could be improved or even cured through a patient discussing feelings and experiences with an analyst. Those who did see bipolar disorder as an actual illness within the brain did not have effective medications that could verify this hunch.

Before the medication revolution, patients were more often committed to hospitals for long or short stays. Typical treatment often included usage of electroshock therapy (ECT). There have been different theories as to how and why ECT works, but the general idea is that chemicals or processes within the brain are jolted out of unproductive and negative patterns. Patients sometimes suffered permanent memory loss, as well as trauma from the experience itself. For quite some time, ECT was more or less discontinued.

However, ECT has made something of a comeback—but usually in the treatment of severe depression, when all other therapies have failed. It also is administered more humanely now. Patients are given anesthesia first, so that they are not conscious during the treatment.

But for bipolar disorder, the advent of lithium and other medications radically altered how bipolar patients were treated. Not surprisingly, this led to a different general sense in society about the disorder. That which is more treatable is less a cause for dread and shame.

 Fact

> A number of famous people are known to have received ECT, including Ernest Hemingway, Vivien Leigh, Gene Tierney, Ken Kesey, Dick Cavett, Michael Moriarity, Tammy Wynette, Lou Reed, Sylvia Plath, and Yves Saint Laurent. For some of these people, ECT was a positive experience, while others spoke of it disparagingly.

Since there is not a magic cure for bipolar disorder, several practical issues surrounding treatment have yet to change. People still must be willing to and actually receive treatment and stay with it. And even if they do receive treatment, other complications can still mitigate its effects. Of those who do seek treatment, there are several subcategories.

Some people find the right treatment, and stay on it. They experience few if any symptoms, and other people would not know they were bipolar unless told.

There also are bipolar patients who experience *many* improvements from medication, but some symptoms seem to be helped more than others. For example, maybe the depression is more under control than the mania. Someone might now be able to concentrate on finishing projects, but still dealing with eating issues. In some cases, episode extremes are kept under control, but the person still feels unable to work or maintain close relationships.

Additionally, people who have multiple disorders often are prescribed a variety of medications. In such instances, the doctor must determine what medications the patient is or is not responding to. And if something seems to go wrong—if the patient has an episode of some sort—perhaps one or more of the medications must be increased or decreased in dosage. Since medications often take at least ten days to start to work—and when they do they might cause upheavals in up or down patterns—patients might well continue to experience at least minor disruptions to their daily routine. For example, about 25 percent of bipolar patients experience increased mania from antidepressants.

L, Essential

Bipolar patients (especially those who have experienced hallucinations) benefit from a magnetic resonance imaging (MRI) or a computerized tomography (CT) scan. These procedures can check for other ailments such as Huntington's disease, brain tumors, and subdural hematomas. Sometimes symptoms attributed to bipolar disorder are caused by some other serious condition.

Additionally, there is the matter of serious side effects. Sometimes a doctor notes that a patient is having side effects from a medication that pose serious health threats, and so takes the patient off that medication. In other instances, patients themselves might state there are serious side effects and insist on going off the medication, even if the doctor does not agree.

Furthermore, some patients fail to respond to medication. There are three more subgroups here—those who never respond to a certain medication, those who respond at first but then fail to do so after a time, and those who start and stop treatment—which disenables it from working.

In these and other ways, treatment has yet to be 100 percent effective. But many types of medications have made enormous differences in people's lives.

Mood Stabilizers

Mood stabilizers are intended to do just what the name says—stop the bipolar mood swings, and bring the individual to a moderate range of thought, behavior, and energy. These drugs seem to work by engaging the neurotransmitters that lie between brain cells. Through a series of chain cellular reactions, the brain-cell membranes are altered in ways that diminish the overstimulation that causes bipolar disorder. The effect is only temporary, however, and so more medication must be taken later that day, or the next day.

Lithium

The first known effective mood stabilizer is still the most frequently prescribed: lithium carbonate, sold under such brand names as Lithane, Lithobid, Lithizine, Lithonate, Lithotabs Duralith, Carbolith, Cibalith-S, and Eskalith. Though the numbers can vary across studies, lithium seems to be effective at least 50 percent of the time, and perhaps as much as 80 percent of the time. Primarily used to stop mania, it has also been shown to have positive effects on depression. It has been approved since the 1970s by the Federal Food and Drug Administration (FDA), and for quite some time had the mania mood-stabilizer market all to itself.

The major drawback to lithium is that it can prove toxic to the kidneys and thyroid, causing coma or even death. However, this rarely happens. More commonly, lithium can cause nausea, diarrhea, skin rashes, weight gain, slurred speech, hand tremor, and muscle twitching and spasms. Other side effects can include drowsiness, memory lapses, an inability to concentrate, and a general sense of apathy. Frequent check-ups with your doctor are needed to make sure that the medication is not only helping you as it should, but is being administered at safe levels for your system. Your doctor should test your blood count, urine, thyroid, and electrolytes before prescribing lithium—or for that matter, any other mood stabilizer.

 ## Fact

Success with lithium is more likely when the patient is not abusing drugs, had a first episode of mania instead of depression, and is not also schizophrenic. A longer history of episodes before treatment is associated with a lower success rate. If one family member responds well to lithium, it is likely that others will as well.

If you are on lithium but go off it for any reason, you should do so gradually, and under a doctor's supervision. Abrupt discontinuance of lithium generally leads to an intense manic episode. There are a number of drugs that can cause the lithium level in your blood system to increase or decrease. If you are taking lithium, you should always make sure that other medications will not interfere with it.

Valproate
A newer type of mood stabilizer, valproate (also known as divalproex, and by brand names such as Epival and Depakote) can reach adequate blood levels more quickly than lithium—and so can stabilize mood more quickly. In fact, it might be more effective at addressing episodes of acute mania than at simple daily maintenance (though it is used both ways). It also might work better on mixed mania, and rapid cycling. It also appears to perform more effectively on patients with neurologic (nervous system) abnormalities, and/or whose manic episodes are known to be especially aggressive. For such people, valproate sometimes works when lithium does not.

Potential side effects can include liver damage, lowered number of blood platelets, and inflammation of the pancreas. Normally, doctors test the patient's blood count regularly, and these serious conditions rarely develop. Less serious side effects can include nausea, drowsiness, problems with concentration, hair loss, increased appetite (and weight gain), and mild tremors. Like lithium, possible negative interactions with other medications should always be considered.

Carbamazepine

On balance, carbamazepine (brand names include Epitol and Tegretol) can help about as many people as lithium or valproate—but once again, the specific people it works best with are slightly different. Carbamazepine has worked well on acute mania, and somewhat less well (though still effectively) with depression. But it tends to work better on patients who also have some schizophrenic symptoms, are rapid cycling, having mixed episodes, or have AD/HD.

The most serious side effect of carbamazepine is that it can lower the white blood-cell counts, as well as the platelet count. It also can increase liver enzyme activity and cause inflammation of the pancreas. But once again, these conditions seldom occur. Older patients have been known to experience abnormal heart rhythms, and difficulty concentrating. Nausea, dizziness, drowsiness, headaches, skin rashes, swelled ankles, and water retention are among the less serious side effects. There are quite a few drugs that carmazepine negatively interacts with.

Other Mood Stabilizers

There are numerous other newer mood stabilizers. Though less tested than older medications, they are all potentially equally effective, and differ mostly in terms of side effects.

Lamotrigine (brand name: Lamictal) has as its most common side effects skin irritation and rash. It also has been associated with nausea, headaches, dizziness, lack of muscle coordination, and both drowsiness and insomnia. Its relatively low side effects are making it a medication of choice, especially when patients have failed to respond to other mood stabilizers. It may be better at controlling rapid cycling and mixed states than valproate or carbamazepine. Besides being used with bipolar patients, it has also been successful with patients with schizophrenia, as well as some patients with unipolar depression, Post-Traumatic Stress Disorder, and Borderline Personality Disorder (when medication is prescribed).

⌷. Essential

Mood stabilizers are often discovered by accident. Lithium was first used as a dissolving agent for another substance that was hoped to be effective in mood stabilizing—but was not. Most of the other current medications were first developed for treating epilepsy. And calcium channel blockers are also used to treat high blood pressure.

Topiramate (Topamax) can cause kidney stones, nausea, decreased appetite (and weight loss), ringing in the ears, and numbness and/or tingling in the feet and hands. It also has been associated with drowsiness, dizziness, and decreased concentration. Probably its most serious side effect is that it has been known to have a boomerang effect on a small number of patients, and actually increase episodic symptoms.

Gabapentin (Nuerontin) has been tested somewhat less, but it appears to have fewer side effects. On a temporary basis, patients might experience dizziness and blurred vision—and so not surprisingly, clumsiness.

Oxcarbazine (Trileptal) contains an oxygen component that diminishes its impact on blood-cell count. However, it may be associated with dizziness and nausea, as well as *hyponatremia*—a lowering of sodium in the blood. This commonly manifests as flu-like symptoms, and swelling of the ankles. However, some patients may find that Trileptal is less powerful than other mood stabilizers.

Calcium Channel Blockers

Though less effective than other kinds of mood stabilizers, calcium channel blockers appear to offer some relief of mania and depression—and sometimes patients who do not respond to other medications have success with these drugs. There are two main varieties: virapamil and nimodipine. The latter tends to work faster. Side effects of these drugs include nausea, dizziness, headache, and low blood pressure.

Antidepressants

Most of the research done on the effectiveness of antidepressants has focused on unipolar, or purely depressed patients. This is because it is easier to measure how well a drug works when there are not other kinds of drugs to consider at the same time—such as mood stabilizers. Hence, not as much is known as could be about which antidepressants are best in treating bipolar disorder. However, one issue that is always considered is the extent to which an antidepressant triggers manic symptoms. Studies indicate that anywhere from one-third to three-fourths of all bipolar patients will have to deal with increases of mania from antidepressants.

The present list of antidepressants includes five general categories.

Selective Serotonin Reuptake Inhibitors (SSRIs)

SSRIs have a success rate of at least 50 percent. They also have a low likelihood of causing mania, and relatively few side effects. This makes them among the most frequently prescribed antidepressants for bipolar patients.

Serotonin is associated with inhibiting depression. SSRIs keep serotonin from being reabsorbed by nerve cells after it has transmitted its impulse. In other words, SSRIs enable the brain to receive and use more serotonin. Familiar varieties of SSRIs include fluoxetine, sertraline, paroxetine, citalopram, and fluvoxamine, better known as Prozac, Zoloft, Paxil, Celexa, and Luvox, respectively.

Many of the side effects associated with SSRIs are familiar from mood stabilizers: nausea, headache, tremors, and both drowsiness and insomnia. SSRIs also are associated with nervousness, sweating, dry mouth, loose bowels, and weight gain. An assortment of these types of symptoms can take the form of *serotonin syndrome*. This means that too much serotonin is in the brain and the nervous system—and that you should tell your doctor, who will probably take you off the medication.

Probably the most widely discussed side effects of SSRIs are sexual in nature. Women experience lowered sex drive, and men often have more difficulty achieving orgasm. Once again, be mindful of possible bad reactions when SSRIs are taken with other prescription drugs.

Monoamine Oxidase Inhibitors (MAOIs)

Monoamine oxidase can increase the likelihood of depression. It exists in two different forms, one of which destroys serotonin, and the other of which destroys dopamine. (The latter is likewise associated with feelings of pleasure, and also plays a role in numerous illnesses such as Parkinson's disease.) The main varieties of these MAOIs— phenelzine (Nardil), and tranylcypromine (Parnate)—inhibit both types of monoamine oxidase. MAOIs are generally not preferred over SSRIs, but nonetheless are often prescribed when patients do not respond to SSRIs or cannot take them.

 Alert

Foods that are off-limits when taking MAOIs include all types of cheese except cream cheese; all pickled or smoked meat, poultry and fish; sausage and salami; chicken and beef liver; fava beans; sauerkraut; and red wine, sherry, and liquors. Fermented products and overripe fruit should also be avoided. MAOIs inhibit the degradation of tyramine—and these foods are high in tyramine.

The side effects associated with MAOIs include drowsiness and insomnia, as well as nervousness, weight gain, transient low blood pressure, and sexual issues. MAOIs also can exacerbate serotonin syndrome. Moreover, when MAOIs are combined with decongestants or other antidepressants, high blood pressure can result. In extreme cases, this can lead to a *hypertensive crisis*, and cause life-threatening conditions such as a stroke.

MAOIs are often a last resort medication used if SSRIs and other kinds of antidepressants have failed to help.

Stimulants

Stimulants are not antidepressants in the strictest sense, but when a patient does not respond to or is unable to take other kinds of antidepressants, a stimulant might be prescribed. Historically, stimulants have popularly been prescribed as appetite suppressants (diet pills). In more recent decades, they have been used to treat AD/HD in children, and in the treatment of narcolepsy, or uncontrollable episodes of sleep. Familiar varieties of stimulants include methylphenidat (Ritalin), dextroamphetamine (Dexedrine), methylphenidate (Methylin), methamphetamine hydrochloride (Desoxyn), and a mixture of amphetamines called Adderall.

These drugs produce a number of side effects, including loss of appetite (and weight), insomnia, headaches, dry mouth, tremors, dizziness, agitation, and increased heart rate and blood pressure. They also have been associated with liver problems, and some people report becoming addicted to them. They furthermore can produce mania or paranoia.

Tricyclic Antidepressants (TCAs)

One of the relative older groups of antidepressants, TCAs are primarily prescribed as a second or third alternative for treating bipolar depression. They work on both serotonin and norepinephrine. Besides often resulting in weight gain, TCAs have been known to increase mania and rapid cycling. Familiar TCAs include Elavil, Normramin, and Vivactil.

Newer Antidepressants

There are a number of new antidepressants developed to work at least as well as SSRIs, with a minimum of side effects.

Bupropion hydrochloride, better known as Wellbutrin, is one such drug. It works not on serotonin, but on dopamine and norapenephrine—another neurotransmitter. Its side effects include insomnia, headaches, constipation, and dry mouth. At exceptionally high levels, it has been associated with seizures. But it also is less likely to produce mania than many other antidepressants, including SSRIs. (This compound, under the name of Zyban, is now also being used to help people quit smoking.) Venlafaxine (Effexor) is similarly effective. However, it addresses levels of serotonin (instead of dopamine) and noropenephrine. At extremely high levels it can result in hypertension. But it has many advantages, including that it works more quickly at attacking depression than many other medications. It is less associated with sexual problems. Its effectiveness is also relatively easy to monitor, as the dosage level seems to correspond clearly with changes in level of depression.

 Fact

Tyramine is a normal body chemical that helps maintain a healthy rate of blood pressure, However, when an MAOI is taken, it can interact with tyramine in a way that causes abnormally high blood pressure. Too much tyramine has also been associated with migraine headaches.

Nephazodone (Serzone) deals with various serotonin-related processes. Nephazodone and Mirtazapine (Remeron), an alpha agonist that works primarily on norepinephrine, both have a sedating effect, which is useful when depression is associated with insomnia or restlessness. However, some patients are uncomfortable with this sedation. Weight gain is a fairly common side effect, but they produce less nausea and work quite rapidly. Both of these newer medications are usually used as a second or third choice. Another new medication is duloxetine (Cymbalta), which is also used to treat physical ailments associated with diabetes. It is an SSNRI, impacting not only levels of serotonin but of norepinephrine as well. Reported side effects have included insomnia and a host of unwelcome mood shifts, including irritability, anxiety, impulsivity, mania and hypomania, and psychomotor restlessness (*akathisia*). Seizures and liver problems might also occur.

Antipsychotics

Antipsychotics are probably best known for being used with schizophrenics. But they also are prescribed when bipolar patients lapse into psychotic symptoms such as hallucinations or delusions. Indeed, these drugs are prescribed to anywhere from 40 to 75 percent of bipolar patients, and probably more than 90 percent of bipolar patients have taken antipsychotics at least once. Many of these newer drugs have also been shown to be effective in treating mania and depression. Drugs used to treat psychosis can be classified by their relative age.

First-Generation Antipsychotics

Also called typical antipsychotics, these drugs were first developed in the 1950s. They are used less often than they used to be, largely because newer drugs seem superior for having fewer side effects. But they still are sometimes used to treat psychosis, and might also be prescribed when patients do not respond to mood stabilizers.

These drugs are either high potency, or low potency. High potency varieties include trifluoperazine (Stelazine), haloperidol (Haldol), fluphenazine decanoate (Prolixin), thiothixene (Navane), and perphenazine (Trilafon). The low-potency types include chlorpromazine (Thorazine), thioridazine (Mellaril), molindone hydrochloride (Moban), loxapine (Loxitane), and mesoridazine besylate (Serentil).

Side effects can include weight gain, seizures, and heart abnormalities. Women might also experience increased appetite, dry mouth, constipation, dry eyes and blurry vision, and sometimes confusion. Taken as a whole in this context, these symptoms are called anticholinergic side effects.

But there are a number of additional problems associated with these typical antipsychotics. These are classified as *extrapyramidal side effects (EPS)*, also called *movement disorder side effects*. EPS can effect upward of 60 percent of the patients on first-generation drugs. Moreover, EPS can take several forms.

Essential

Antipsychotics are also used to help people get down off of bad acid trips. That is because the hallucinations and distortions produced by hallucinogens such as LSD mimic psychotic delusions. In fact, laboratory rats are sometimes injected with LSD in order to then test for the effectiveness of antipsychotic drugs.

Parkinsonian EPS is aptly named, in that the symptoms replicate those of Parkinson's disease. These include muscle stiffness, slowed speech and movement, and tremors. Many of the same drugs used to treat Parkinson's disease are prescribed in these instances.

Tardive dyskinesia (TD) usually occurs after being on typical antipsychotics for long periods of time. It is probably the most visible kind of EPS, and thus the most troubling for the patient. It involves involuntary and repetitive twisting movements of body muscles—including those of the face, limbs, and trunk. Facially, people thus afflicted might blink, chew, or move their lips and tongue uncontrollably.

Acute dystonic reactions are somewhat less severe muscle spasms of the neck, face, and tongue. These symptoms are most commonly seen in younger male patients.

Akethisia is experienced in the legs as a restless need to keep walking or pacing.

Neuroleptic malignant syndrome (NMS) is much less common, but extremely serious. If present, not only should antipsychotic medication cease, but there should be immediate medical treatment. The symptoms include an elevated white blood-cell count, fever, severe rigidity of muscles, confusion, and unstable blood pressure, breathing, and heart rate.

Second-Generation Antipsychotics

Also called atypical antipsychotics, these newer drugs are associated with both better treatment of psychosis and lessened presence of EPS. All of these drugs may be associated with arrhythmias of the heart, so regular EKGs are recommended.

Clozapine (also called Closzaril) is one of the oldest atypical antipsychotics. It has been shown to be effective in treating manic symptoms, in addition to psychotic ones, in around 50 percent of patients who have tried it. However, given the side effects associated with it, it generally is not recommended as a substitute for mood stabilizers unless patients have not responded to them.

Clozapine has several temporary side effects, including drooling, lack of control of urinary functions, and the anticholinergic side effects outlined above. Over a longer period of time, there can be significant weight gain, elevation in cholesterol and tryglycerides, and inflammation of the pancreas or heart muscle. Sometimes, patients have experienced seizures as well. Perhaps the most serious side effect is a drop in the white blood-cell count. Patients therefore are required to get blood counts performed on a regular basis—especially during the first months of treatment. Numerous other drugs should be avoided due to negative interactions.

A somewhat more recent medication is risperidone, or Risperdal. It seems to treat a wide range of bipolar symptoms (including mania and depression) in over 50 percent of those tested. Common side effects include sleepiness, dizziness, abnormal body temperature, increased appetite or weight gain, and (in rare cases) prolonged and painful erection in males. Older patients, or patients with other brain ailments, might experience EPS. It also might exacerbate mania in some patients.

Olanzepine, or Zyprexa, is a newer antipsychotic, and has been shown to also have a positive effect on mania, though possibly of the more mild variety. Once again, weight gain is an issue, as is cholesterol and triglyceride levels. It also has been associated with EPS. Moreover, it might lead to certain forms of diabetes. Other side effects can include sleepiness, dizziness, and dry mouth.

 Fact

The newer, atypical antipsychotic drugs have been considered as significant a breakthrough for schizophrenic patients as lithium and other mood stabilizers were for bipolar patients. Like mood stabilizers, these newer antipsychotics do not work for everyone all of the time. But approximately 60 percent of the schizophrenic patients who use them have successful results.

Quetiapine, or Seroquel, likewise has been used to treat a wide range of manic-depressive symptoms. It has a relatively low incidence of EPS. Side effects include weight gain, increased cholesterol and tryglyceride levels, nausea, dry mouth, dizziness, and postural hypotension (dizziness or light-headedness upon standing, or fainting).

Ziprasidone, or Geodon, is an extremely new atypical antipsychotic. It seems to be effective in treating both psychotic distortions and depression. There is less weight gain associated with it than other atypical antipsychotics.

Anti-Anxiety Drugs and Sleep Aids

In addition to medications that treat the primary symptoms of bipolar disorder, there are other drugs that can aid in episodes of relatively minor anxiety, and also help the patient to sleep. Many non-bipolar people also use these medications. For the bipolar person, these drugs might help to remove the remaining rough edges of someone's condition. At the same time, they should be prescribed with caution, as some can be quite addictive.

Benzodiazepines

Benzodiazepines are a familiar class of drugs commonly prescribed for conditions such as anxiety and insomnia. They often are given to patients before major surgery, and are used to treat a range of psychic injuries and mental and behavioral problems associated with anxiety. At one time, these drugs also were prescribed fairly often to treat mania. Now, they are more likely to be used by bipolar patients for short-term use only, to help treat the anxiety or sleeplessness that might accompany acute mania. When used for this purpose, these drugs usually supplement other medications.

Common forms of benzodiazepines include diazepam (Valium), chlordiazepoxide (Librium), alprazolam (Xanax), lorazepam (Activan), triazolam (Halcion), and clonazepam (Klonopin). (The lattermost might be prescribed temporarily, until mood stabilizers have taken effect.) Besides being highly addictive, these drugs have been associated with drowsiness and memory loss. Persons taking these drugs are often advised not to operate complex machinery. They should also not be taken with alcohol.

These drugs also are associated with diminished inhibitions. This means that patients who are especially prone to extreme behaviors—including suicide—should be given these drugs on a limited basis at the most.

Sleep Aids

All people benefit from a good night's sleep. But for a person with bipolar disorder, not being able to sleep can signal the possibility of an episode. Mood stabilizers, in dealing with mania, might enable patients to get a normal night's sleep. But if insomnia is still an issue—or if it is being caused by one of the medications—a doctor might prescribe a sleeping aid. These come from a class of drugs called *hypnotics*. They temporarily alter certain processes in the brain that may be the cause of insomnia. Often, these drugs are prescribed for short-term or sporadic use, as it is possible to develop a dependency on them. Withdrawal symptoms can include seizures, increased heart rate, nausea, abdominal cramps, tremors, and anxiety. Regular usage can lead to impairment of memory and other cognitive functions. In some cases, these medications can cause hallucinations.

Eszopiclone, or Lunesta, is a newer drug that is associated with far fewer side effects: dizziness, drowsiness, and issues of coordination. People with liver disease will need to at least start with low dosages. Importantly, it does not appear to become less effective over time, and so can be prescribed for long-term use. (That is to say, there may be fewer addiction issues associated with it.)

At present, two other prescription drugs tend to be relatively less likely to cause serious side effects (though they still can do so). They therefore are prescribed fairly often, albeit for short-term use only.

Zolpidem, or Ambian, is an imidzopyridine. While there can be withdrawal symptoms, they are somewhat less likely to occur, or to be less intense, than with older types of sleep aids. And while it can be habit-forming, this again happens relatively less than with older drugs. It generally appears to work safely with SSRIs. In some cases, it causes depression and/or insomnia.

Zelaplon, or Sonata, appears to have even milder side effects—though yet again, some people have strong adverse reactions. One of the benefits of this medication is that it can be taken in the middle of the night. That is to say, if you try sleeping without it but cannot—or awaken in the middle of the night—you can take Sonata, and still wake up at a desired time feeling refreshed.

Older sleep aids are also still prescribed on occasion. These include temazepam (Restoril) and desyrel (Trazodone). The former is a benzodiazapine. Side effects include headache, nausea, drowsiness, nervousness, dry mouth, and loss of equalibrium. Trazadone might be prescribed when insomnia is drug-induced. It also has been used to treat depression and physical ailments.

There also are over-the-counter sleep aids. Though these of course do not require a prescription, you should consult your doctor about taking them, in the event that so doing would conflict with other treatment matters. These medications include melatonin (often available in health food stores), which is a hormone produced in the pineal gland during sleep. Other benzodiazepines have also been shown to aid in sleep in some patients. These medications can cause tremors or increased heart rate, vomiting, dizziness, blurred vision, problems with concentration, and difficulties with urination.

 Alert

Another common side effect of benzodiazepines is clumsiness and falling down. In fact, people taking this class of drug are 40 to 70 percent more likely to fracture a hip, depending upon the strength of the dosage taken.

Finding the Right Medication(s)

Bipolar disorder will likely mean treatment consisting of several medications. This means the doctor must find a way to treat all these symptoms in harmony. Some of the likely issues that your doctor will keep in mind in prescribing medication include:

- The known interactions that occur with the various bipolar medications
- The known interactions that occur with any other medications that the patient must take regularly, as well as the patient's medical history
- Regular (and honest) reports from the patient regarding both improvement and side effects
- The need for maximum inclusiveness, with a minimum of redundancy

This last point means that the doctor will want to treat as many symptoms as possible, while at the same time not prescribing more medication than needed. For example, a doctor probably would not prescribe two mood stabilizers, or two antidepressants, unless there were problems with responding to only one of each.

Some patients are luckier than others. There are those who respond highly favorably to the first medication(s) prescribed. They will still need to get regular check-ups, but the bipolar symptoms themselves seem largely under control.

Other patients might experience harmful side effects, or not respond to a given medication, and so an alternate is prescribed. And perhaps this alternate sets in motion further changes in the medication regime, given that the new drug used to treat depression (for example) might be better combined with a different mood stabilizer.

Also, it is reasonable to expect *some* side effects. In other words, do not let dry mouth, for example, lead you to conclude you should go off a certain medication, if it otherwise is working as it should. Remember that *everyone* suffers from minor malfunctions of the body sometimes, and many people adjust even to permanent changes in bodily conditions. Going off of medication hardly guarantees that you will never again experience nausea or headaches. Only serious side effects that might permanently impede your health and well-being should generally be considered in deciding to switch medications. And of course, the decision should be made in consultation with a doctor.

CHAPTER 7

Additional Methods for Dealing with Bipolar

Since bipolar disorder involves physiological processes within the brain, it follows that medication that alters these processes would be highly effective. But medication may not be all that is needed. Acting out mania and depression can be disorienting to self and others—and sometimes quite frightening. There are a number of other kinds of steps that can be taken to help ensure that the bipolar person and his loved ones are able to have normal, happy lives.

When Medication Is Not Enough

If you are bipolar, medication is the foundation for a happy life—but you will still have to build on top of it. Here are some of the key areas that will need to be addressed. One important area to work on is coming to terms with the past. Medication cannot magically erase the complicated feelings that emerge around bipolar disorder. Obviously, there are still many issues to be sorted out.

In the throes of a manic or depressive episode, a person with bipolar says or does many things that seem senseless, destructive, or thoughtless to the onlooker—and to the self, once medicated. There probably are people in one's life that are entitled to a sincere discussion, sometimes even an apology. This includes forgiveness within the self, and some deep thinking about where you have been, and where you are headed.

A bipolar person, as well as loved ones, will also benefit from fully accepting the diagnosis. Some people react with relief at being told they are bipolar—that there *is* an explanation for all that has been happening. Others might respond with disbelief. But in either case, there is the reality of medication, regular check-ups, and other special needs that will need to be faced . . . for the rest of the patient's life. This type of acceptance might require changing a lot of assumptions about who you are.

Acceptance also means accepting the possibility of future episodes. Understanding bipolar disorder means understanding that it is something that does not just go away. A favorable response to medication means nothing if a patient stops treatment. Some patients do not respond to medication as well as others, and find their symptoms *diminished* but still something they must contend with.

Yet at the same time, it is important to cultivate self-confidence. Getting diagnosed bipolar is a serious matter, but it is *not* a death sentence. Many bipolar people accomplish extraordinary things; many also live perfectly normal and fulfilling lives. Still others might be somewhat limited in what they can do even with medication, but manage to find worthwhile activities in a given day of life. You need to find a way to accept being bipolar, and still be happy to face a new day.

 Fact

The General Social Survey (GSS) is administered to a random sample of the U.S. population. It includes questions about personal happiness. However, some sources note that the survey is administered in the spring—the time of year in which moods tend to be at their highest. Thus, some have wondered if GSS people tend to overstate their degree of personal happiness.

Like anyone else, it is also good to work at having a healthy body, along with a healthy mind. All people are happier when they are healthy, both inside and out. You owe it to yourself to not only have your mind in a happy place, but also to see that you are eating right and staying fit. More to the point, it will be much harder to feel happy when your body is full of complaints. And there even is some evidence that certain foods can help in building healthy cells.

In these and other ways, getting "well" can mean much more than simply finding the right medication. Though medication makes wellness possible, the rest is up to you.

Finding the Right Therapy

If you want to come to terms with your past, and have a good sense about your future, you might decide that in addition to taking medication from a psychiatrist you should also see a therapist. It's important to recognize that there are different kinds of therapy. These are not just different styles depending on the individual therapist, but actual different schools of thought on how to best treat patients.

Analytic Psychotherapy

Popularized by Freud and others, analytic psychotherapy is based on the idea that your personality was formed on the basis of past events. Specifically, it contends that all children pass through certain phases of development. These phases are marked by a conflict between the self's desire for pleasure (the *id*), and the voice of society, which demands conformity (the *superego*). The *ego* is the part of the self that then tries to mitigate between the two. A healthy ego finds constructive solutions. But a damaged ego will give in too often to either the id or the superego. How healthy the ego is depends upon the early experiences of the self in regard to the parents. Thus, how the parents nurture the child plays a major role in who someone becomes as an adult. Someone who is not fully developed as an adult is seen as needing to relive these childhood dramas that are holding him back.

In this therapeutic framework, you should expect to delve deeply into your past. You will do most of the talking yourself, in order to arrive at your own truth about the patterns in your life. The therapist will encourage you to understand how present situations reflect unresolved feelings from your past—especially your childhood. To explore those parts of yourself that are buried and unknown to you, you also might be encouraged to explore the meanings of your dreams, or why you have such a strong reaction to certain situations. Much of this work is called *free association*. In theory, this type of therapy is conducted several times a week for five to seven years, but in actual practice it might be less often per week, and for fewer or more years.

If you want to sort out how you were misunderstood as a child, or how the ways you were raised might have exacerbated your bipolar symptoms, you might find analytic psychotherapy useful.

Behavioral Therapy

Behaviorism was founded by people such as B. F. Skinner and John Watson. These scientists believed that it was impossible to know the self the way someone like Freud claimed. People could not really know or understand their inner drives, but what *could* be known and understood was actual behavior. For the behaviorist, a patient can be judged as getting better or worse on the basis of observable behavior—the things the patient says and does. It does not matter why the patient changes patterns of behavior, only that change actually happens. Change in behavior occurs through a system of *punishment* and *rewards*. Undesired behavior is punished and made *extinct*, while desired behavior is rewarded and is *reinforced*.

In concert with the therapist (and possibly with loved ones), you will be encouraged to develop strategies for rewarding desired behavior, and punishing undesired behavior. To use a simple example, if you have trouble finishing projects, you can develop a way of rewarding yourself for each step you complete.

If you want to break certain bad habits and replace them with more productive ones, behavioral therapy might be good for you.

Cognitive Therapy

A number of famous thinkers have contributed to cognitive psychology, including Noam Chomsky and George Miller. From the cognitive perspective, behavior and emotion come from thoughts. People make certain choices in their daily lives on the basis of what they perceive about life or themselves. If people tend to do destructive things—if they are easy to anger, for example, or do not permit themselves much pleasure—it is because their thoughts and beliefs need to be changed. Patients in cognitive therapy are therefore encouraged to look at situations with fresh eyes. Rather than assume that So-and-So doesn't like them, or that *nobody* does, or that this person is bad and that situation is awful, patients are trained to consider different, more constructive ideas. Empathy for others, and affirmations for the self, might be some of the areas covered. Patients might learn to think of things less in black-and-white terms, and embrace more of the gray area of life.

Ⅼ Essential

In a cognitive therapeutic setting, you might be given affirmations to remind yourself to think differently about certain situations. Progress is apparent when you start to genuinely respond differently to certain kinds of situations. When something no longer upsets you the way it would have in the past because you are thinking about it differently, unproductive behavioral patterns can be broken. (Cognitive Therapy and Behavioral Therapy are sometimes used in concert as Cognitive Behavioral Therapy.)

If being bipolar has led you to form deeply ingrained assumptions about yourself and other people, you might gain from cognitive therapy.

Humanistic Therapy

Popularized by Carl Rogers, humanistic therapy examines how someone feels a sense of purpose in life—by learning to live a life of purpose. The emphasis is often on teaching people greater tolerance and compassion for their fellow humans, and becoming socially involved citizens. The remedy to personal unhappiness is seen as having a goal in life that can benefit other people. In this way, one's life takes on a deeper meaning, and everyday challenges do not overwhelm.

Within this type of framework, your will be encouraged to look at the proverbial "big picture." Does your life seem to mean anything, and if not, what can you do to make a difference—to make the world a better place to live in? If you can feel like a productive citizen, you may find that many of your other problems or issues seem far less important. (In Chapter 15, specific suggestions are offered as to how you can improve the social conditions for bipolar people and the mentally ill as a whole.)

If you are a bipolar person looking for a way to help other people and feel that your life has a deeper purpose, humanistic therapy could be what you need.

Jungian Therapy

Carl Jung was a student of Freud's who eventually developed a different approach to mental wellness. Jungian therapy places great emphasis upon creativity and imagination. Life is viewed as a kind of story, with characters, a plot, and symbolic meanings. According to Jung, there is a *collective unconscious* that informs our impressions of life, and we use these shared symbolic meanings to understand ourselves and others.

Jungian therapists often encourage patients to view their lives in a highly creative and imaginative manner. For example, if your write or paint, you might share your stories or artwork with the therapist to uncover meanings about your nature. You also might be encouraged to approach your problems within a storybook-like framework in which you are the "hero" and the various people you encounter in your journey provide you with what you need to achieve your goals. Even people who seem to be negative influences or obstacles might be opportunities to make you braver or wiser, or give you something else that you need to complete the journey.

If you want to join the list of bipolar people with a rich creative life, the Jungian approach to self-understanding might be a useful tool.

Of course, there also are therapists who combine different approaches. In fact, many do. Still, it never hurts to ask a potential therapist what school(s) of thought he or she draws upon. Also important to consider is your basic connection to the therapist: Is this someone that you feel comfortable sharing with? Do you feel the therapist really hears what you have to say, or not?

Therapies Beyond the Inner Self

Besides working on your thoughts and behaviors per se, you should strongly consider other kinds of therapeutic settings that potentially can help you in the wider range of your life.

Couples and family therapy is just what it sounds like—opportunities to be in therapy with your spouse and/or other family members to sort out your collective issues as a couple or family. A variety of techniques might be used, but a basic goal is often to improve communication within the couple or family. Strategies and skills are provided to enable each person involved to truly *listen* to the other(s). Oftentimes, people in close relations assume they already know how the other person or persons feel, or why certain actions occurred. But in these kinds of therapeutic settings, such assumptions are set aside in order to let all concerned speak their own truth. There also might be suggestions for how to better handle certain kinds of situations as they arise, and what other kinds of activities might make everyone feel closer.

 Fact

Roughly 50 percent of all Americans claim to experience a serious psychological problem at least once, and nearly two-thirds think that professional help should be sought in such instances. Upward of 60 percent of all employee absences are due to psychological factors. However, less than 30 percent of people in the United States will actually seek professional help.

Group therapy usually consists of a small number of people who all have a particular condition or goal in common. For example, perhaps you can be in a therapy group consisting of bipolar patients. These groups have a therapist who facilitates, posing questions and offering up group exercises. The group therapist also facilitates comments between group members. Oftentimes, the patients in the group can make suggestions to each other, as well as ask each other questions or perhaps even challenge one another to arrive at a deeper truth. One of the facilitator's jobs here is to make sure these kinds of discussions are productive and helpful. Particularly if you have trouble relating to other people, you might find group therapy helpful. (See also support groups below.)

Occupational therapy is available to people with serious mental conditions, as well as people who have experienced profound physical injuries, or who have terminal illnesses. The occupational therapist will work with the patient to find strategies for independent living and maximizing their general well-being. People who might otherwise need to be hospitalized or under intense medical care can find ways of taking care of themselves, instead. The therapist might visit the patient within a professional medical setting, a school, or at the patient's home.

Vocational training might also prove useful. This provides training (and sometimes certification) in a particular career. If you need to learn a new or different kind of job skill, or have been out of work for some time but would like to try again, you might consider vocational training. There are many public and private programs available to teach people new job skills.

Diet and Exercise

An old saying posits that if you do not have your health, you do not have anything. As previously discussed, poor health can lead to medicines that conflict with bipolar medications, or feelings of general discomfort that might help set in motion a bipolar episode. However, since bipolar people often need to learn more about moderation, it is important not to go from one extreme to another.

Diet

It is unrealistic for most people to try to live without *any* guilty indulgences when it comes to food. Moreover, for the bipolar person, a fanatical eating lifestyle can be associated with undesired behavior. It is best to avoid extremes, even when it comes to diet and nutrition.

Fortunately, it is the law of the land for food products to be labeled with nutritional information. Thus, before you eat something, you can look on the label to see what it does or does not contain. *Always pay attention to how many servings there are.* Some food producers try to fool the consumer by taking, say, one ounce of food and dividing it up into ten servings. Thus, a food that eaten in total has 1,000 calories might "seem" to only have a 100, because you misread the label.

Food properties to be aware of include:

- **Calories:** Depending on what your doctor tells you, you probably want no more than about 2,000 calories a day.
- **Fats:** In moderation, fats are important to a daily diet. Certain nutrients are fat soluble, meaning that without fats you will not get all the nutrients your body needs. On average, about 25 to 30 percent of a daily calorie intake should be fats. Five grams of fat equals one teaspoon.
- **Sodium:** No more than 2,300 milligrams a day is generally considered healthy.
- **Cholesterol:** Usually, less than 300 milligrams a day is acceptable.
- **Fiber:** Two grams of fiber per serving is considered good, and five or more grams makes a food high fiber.
- **Sugar:** If there is no fruit in the serving, four grams or less is considered healthy. Foods with fruit in them can go as high as eight grams per serving.

There are a number of snack foods that contain at least some healthy ingredients. These can include: almonds, pumpkin and sunflower seeds, dried fruits, trail mix, granola bars, nutrition bars, baked chips and crackers, bottled fruit or vegetable juices (better without extra sweeteners), and milk and milk alternatives, such as soy.

Supplements

Several natural sources contribute to the growth of healthy cells—which once again can only help. These include omega-3, or polyunsaturated fatty acids found in meat and oily fish; and inositol, a natural supplement. (Some research indicates that bipolar and schizophrenic people are naturally lacking in fatty acids.) Furthermore, foods high in amino acids are rich in tryptophan, a natural relaxant. Dairy, soy, eggs, seafood, poultry, meats, whole grains, beans, hazelnuts, peanuts, and sesame and sunflower seeds are all high in amino acids.

L. Essential

Besides being found in capsule form at your local health food store, inositol is found in the human eye and heart. In helping with healthy cell production, it also has been reported to have positive effects regarding male hair loss, eczema, constipation, unhealthy estrogen levels, and high cholesterol.

Also, Saint John's wort is promoted as a natural antidote to depression. It can often be found in health food stores, or vitamin sections in drug stores or supermarkets. Research suggests some modest findings of support in cases of mild depression—it is a mild form of SRI (serotonin reuptake inhibitor, as per Chapter 6). While there is little hard evidence to suggest it is effective in cases of major depression, bipolar patients might consider using it as a supplement. Saint John's wort can produce relatively minor side effects in some people, and it also might cause an adverse reaction when combined with other antidepressants. It also might produce mania, and since it is not regulated by the Food and Drug Administration (FDA), its full range of side effects has not been determined. You should consult your doctor before taking it. A few other herbal remedies (such as ginkgo, valerian, and kava) have also been promoted as natural anti-depressants, though there is even less data available on them.

On balance, it is possible to pay attention to diet without becoming fanatical about it. With a moderate attitude, the bipolar person can eat well and still have some occasional indulgences like anyone else.

Exercise

Exercise can take many forms. Increasingly, people think "exercise" is something that requires a costly gym membership—indoors. But simply walking outside in the fresh air is also exercise. Even just thirty minutes of walking a day can improve your heart rate, your muscle tone, and your disposition. If you take public transportation to work, you can get on and off a stop or two early, to add a few more minutes of walking to your day. Or if you drive to work, you can likewise park a short distance from your destination. Being in the fresh air and sun-shine—even in cold weather—can have positive effects on depression, and can sometimes have a calming effect on hyperactivity.

Also, do not discount alternative forms of exercise, such as yoga. Many people find yoga to be both relaxing and invigorating, and some research suggests that regular yoga breathing exercises can aid in depression and anxiety.

Perhaps the single most important factor in finding a workable exercise regime is picking something you enjoy doing. It is not likely that you will stick to an exercise program that you do not enjoy—particularly if you are bipolar, and therefore often easily distracted. If music makes exercise more fun, do not forget to play your favorite music. Talk to your doctor about how much and what kinds of exercise might prove the most beneficial, and think creatively.

Support Groups

Adjusting to the reality of bipolar disorder can be easier if you remember that you are not alone. And there is probably no better way of being reminded of this than by being part of a support group. Besides being in an atmosphere in which you need not worry about being "different," there will be stories from others that might comfort, inform, or inspire you. There also is the possibility of forming friendships with people who will understand what you are going through.

Bipolar Disorder Groups

Your doctor, hospital, and public library are some of the resources you might contact for finding a nearby support group that exclusively deals with bipolar disorder. The Depression and Bipolar Support Alliance is another great resource. Visit the DBSA Web site at *www.dbsalliance.org*.

Groups focused specifically on bipolar disorder are normally run by a trained facilitator and can take three basic forms:

- **Groups for bipolar people only:** The main purpose of a support group is to provide hope and understanding based on shared needs and experiences—as opposed to necessarily altering thoughts or behavioral patterns. A support group does not necessarily have a trained therapist facilitating; the members of the group might take turns leading the meeting.
- **Groups for bipolar people's loved ones:** The emphasis is often on learning better coping strategies and cognitive skills in dealing with a bipolar person—who may or may not be in treatment. There also will probably be an atmosphere in which people can share both hope and sorrow regarding their loved one.
- **Groups for both bipolar people and their loved ones:** Some support groups bring together both the bipolar person and those who are close to him. The emphasis is often on sharing thoughts and feelings in ways that build trust and understanding between the bipolar person and his family.

More General Groups

If there is not a bipolar support group within a reasonable distance of your home, there might be a more general support group about other mental or mood disorders, or about these disorders in general. You might even find affinity within a 12-Step group such as Al-Anon, which provides support for the family and friends of alcoholics. (As noted elsewhere, bipolar people often develop issues with alcohol and substance abuse.) There are other 12-Step programs that you also might find useful. However, it is important to keep in mind that some people in 12-Step groups advocate being medication-free. Beyond this, there might even be a general support group for people with troubled spouses, children, or parents.

 Fact

> There certainly is nothing unusual in people turning to other people for major help or support. In fact, around 40 percent of the U.S. population will participate in some type of voluntary or support group over the course of a lifetime. Whether as a helper or a person in need—or both—you are part of a much larger trend.

If there are no known support groups in your general vicinity that seem useful to you, there is still another possibility: Talk to your doctor about starting one up. And in today's world, the Internet is yet another resource. E-mail groups and online chat rooms are available on a variety of topics and issues. You might try going to online links such as: *www.supportpath.com.*

Integrating Spirituality

"Spirituality" can mean many things. It can mean becoming active in an organized religion. But it can also mean pursuing more loosely structured, non-denominational spiritual activities through groups or books.

Furthermore, it can mean an attitude—a generalized belief that there is rhyme and reason to being alive. Some people feel spiritual being in nature, looking up at the stars, or listening to their favorite music.

Whatever form it takes, some sort of spiritual orientation might prove helpful in learning to live with bipolar disorder. (It is *not* a requirement, but again, it might help.) Perhaps you need to feel a deeper purpose about who you are, given that you or someone you care about is bipolar. Or maybe you need to feel that bipolar disorder is about something more than neurotransmitters and genetics, that in some deep way, there is a reason for why it has been brought into your life.

 Alert

The key word here is integrating spirituality. There is nothing wrong with believing in powers greater than humankind, and good can even come from such beliefs. However, bipolar people must first and foremost seek out a medical treatment that works for them. Many organized religions or informal spiritual practices are accommodating to the realities of bipolar disorder, but some are not.

In general, you should avoid spiritual groups or practices that advocate that bipolar disorder can be "cured" through non-medical means. This can include mental exercises, strong prayer, faith healing, exorcising a demon, or somehow atoning to God or "working through karma." These alternatives are dubious at best and can lead to unfortunate consequences when the bipolar person not only suffers a relapse but is made to feel weak or ashamed for having "failed" to change the circumstance.

There are some groups that not only claim that bipolar disorder can be "cured" through this alternate means, but that it is the only way it should be dealt with. These groups might go so far as to coerce a bipolar person to *not* take medications, but to instead rely solely on the group and its belief systems. This is taking things to an even more dangerous extreme. Moreover, the new religious zeal the person displays upon being "cured" might actually be an undiagnosed episode of mania.

It might very well be that ours is an overly medicated society, and that people often turn too quickly to pills for a solution when they would be better off changing their behavior or looking inside themselves. But when a group of people insists that nobody should ever use medication for anything, this group is being at best naïve, and can cause tragic outcomes.

Getting Help with Other Problems

You might feel very optimistic when you respond well to medication, as well as when your family and friends are supportive and understanding. But being bipolar can still cause problems, no matter how effective medication is. And things that have nothing to do with being bipolar can—and will—go wrong. Surprisingly, even excessively good news might make for problems where bipolar disorder is concerned. For example, ringing in the spirit of celebration can set in motion mood instability or feelings of grandiosity.

Dealing with Loss

For a bipolar person, a major loss, such as that of a loved one through death or divorce, or loss of a job, can certainly make depression—or sometimes even mania—a strong possibility. Depending on the nature of the loss, there might also be a tendency to become overly involved in other people's lives. Or perhaps the person will seek comfort through inappropriate sex.

Essentially, there are three main sources you can turn to in dealing with profound loss. The first is professional support. Honesty is extremely important in seeking help from a doctor. Do not say you are "fine" when you are hurting. Instead, ask for help; inquire if more medication would be appropriate. If you are seeing a therapist, request an extra session if you feel you truly need it. If you start engaging in behavior that is associated with a symptom of bipolar disorder—such as radically changing eating or sleeping patterns, spending lots of money, or having random and excessive sex—you need to inform the doctor or doctors that you deal with.

There also is personal support; your larger support system can be extremely important, whether loved ones or a support group. Share how you feel. If others are touched by the loss as well, listen as they share in return. At the same time, remember that the people in your support network have other needs and responsibilities to attend to. They will try to be there for you as much as they can be, but they may well have to go to work or care for other loved ones. Also, avoid getting overly gossipy about whatever just happened. If you have obsessive thoughts about what other people did or should be doing, share them with your doctor.

 ## Fact

Anywhere from 50 to 70 percent of the appointments made with primary physicians in a given year prove to not have any physical basis. Instead, these ailments would seem to be psychological in origin—people dealing with loss or upheavals in relatively ineffective ways.

A third resource is self-support. Within yourself, try to remember that loss is a part of life. Positive new beginnings often get set in motion because of something that has seemingly gone "wrong." Perhaps there are books or affirmations that can help you to remember this. If you have a spiritual foundation, this might also provide comfort or insight.

Dealing with Gain

Many people fear change—even positive change. There is a tendency to get used to things as they are, and so people sometimes turn down major opportunities just because they would rather not have to make such a dramatic adjustment. For a bipolar person who has found a daily routine that works, new opportunities can be that much more unsettling. Moving to a new area can mean having to find a new doctor. A promotion or increase in finances can mean new responsibilities that complicate one's life. There can be mania and grandiosity—or, if one fails, the possibility of depression.

If you are succeeding professionally, or if someone important has come into your life, the same basic strategies should be employed. Tell your doctor(s) how this new development is making you think and behave. Share with your loved ones—once again, in a healthy moderation. And in private moments with yourself, remember that loss and sadness will come your way again—that neither good news nor bad news lasts forever. Feel deserving of your good fortune, but remember that there are other people who are likewise deserving of good fortune, and you are no "better" or "worse" than they are.

CHAPTER 8

What Happens Without Treatment?

If everyone who was bipolar was able to receive the right medical treatment for their manic and depressive symptoms, bipolar disorder itself would be much less of a problem than it is. However, the sad truth is that some people never receive the right medical treatment—or receive medical treatment at all. This chapter presents some of the reasons why this happens, as well as some of the statistics on the tragic results that all too commonly follow.

Suicide and Bipolar: The Tragic Facts

Many people do not realize that suicide is one of the leading causes of death—both in the United States and around the world. Rightfully, there is a great deal of activity to find cures for various deadly ailments. But it could be argued that not nearly enough attention is given to finding ways of stopping suicide. Since technically suicide is a self-inflicted act, many people assume there is nothing much that society can do. But if one considers that diagnosable mood disorders are often the cause of suicide—and that these disorders are often treatable—funding to stop suicide can seem not so different from funding to stop cancer or AIDS.

Global Suicide Rates

Globally, suicide rates have increased by as much as 60 percent over the past half a century. Today, suicide is the second leading cause of death for women between the ages of fifteen and forty-four. It is the fourth leading cause of death for men in the same age group—war being right behind at number five. Worldwide each year, about 7 percent of the deaths of men and women in this age group are caused by suicide. Taking all age groups into account, suicide causes about 2 percent of the world's deaths. This means that about 6 million people a year take their lives.

 Fact

As much as one half of all bipolar people will attempt suicide at least once. In the United States alone, this means that somewhere between 1 and 2½ million bipolar people will attempt suicide, and between 50,000 and 75,000 of them will succeed. And untreated patients are at least twice as likely to both try and succeed at taking their own lives.

Despite many differences in culture, globally about 90 percent of all suicides and suicide attempts involve mental disorders. Other factors play a vital role, such as the extent of social support; not all people with mental problems kill themselves. But there is no denying that whatever other situations are involved, mental illness is key to understanding suicide.

Suicide in the United States

In the United States, about 35,000 people commit suicide a year— or about one suicide every twenty minutes. It is the eighth leading cause of death across age groups. There are 1.5 times more suicides each year than homicides. Twice as many people die from suicide than from AIDS.

About three times as many males die of suicide than females, though females are three times more likely to attempt it. The method used seems to account for some of the number differences. Males use firearms about 60 percent of the time, which is a more effective method than those preferred by women (pills and razors). In fact, the annual number of suicides by firearms usually more or less matches the total number of homicides. As it happens, about three-fourths of the men who commit suicide are white.

Probably upward of 700,000 attempt suicide. Over 130,000 people are hospitalized each year for attempting suicide, and about another 120,000 are treated in emergency centers.

Suicide and Youth

The rates of suicide are rising rapidly among youth. Various studies on international suicide rates have estimated that the rates have increased by as much as 300 percent over the past fifty years. In one-third of the countries around the world, youth are now the highest at-risk group for suicide. More teenagers die by their own hand each year than from heart ailments, AIDS, cancer, or other diseases combined. In the United States suicide is now the third leading cause of death among people aged fifteen to twenty-four—or about 4,000 people each year.

The reasons for this rapid increase in numbers include:

- **Puberty arriving at a younger age:** This means a higher percentage of people than ever deal with non-childhood issues and dilemmas.
- **Higher rates of mood disorder:** The onslaught of puberty at an earlier age can mean more young adults afflicted by mood disorder.
- **Higher rates of substance abuse:** Substance abuse exacerbates mood disorder.

In sum, bipolar disorder is absolutely related to climbing rates of suicide. Patients who do not get treatment are in a serious state of risk.

Other Risk Factors

Besides suicide, the untreated bipolar person is especially vulnerable to a number of violent and troubling scenarios, such as homicide. About 10 percent of the homicides committed each year have a perpetrator with a serious mental disorder such as bipolar. About another 10 percent of mentally ill people injure another person, and yet another 10 percent threaten to.

The grandiosity that emerges from mania can make someone feel unquestionably right. It also can seem as though nothing bad can happen to the self, and that everything one does is perfection. Since there also can be strong feelings of mistrust toward others, it follows that an extreme manic episode can make the taking of someone's life seem appropriate, perhaps even necessary. Certainly acts of violence and destruction are common to manic episodes.

At the same time, the mentally ill are probably twice as likely to be victims of homicide. In the case of bipolar people, perhaps there is a family member who simply feels pushed beyond limits. In the midst of wild, manic accusations, or sudden, deep depression, someone is murdered, out of frustration, by someone she knows.

 Alert

Depression can make life seem meaningless and without dimension. Therefore, an afflicted person can see it as "logical"—perhaps even "humane"—to take someone else's life. Moreover, since untreated bipolar disorder can cause outright hallucinations and distortions, it becomes all the more likely that someone might commit homicide.

In addition to suicide and homicide, there are a number of general risks associated with bipolar disorder when left untreated. For example, in an effort to deal with their symptoms on their own, probably at least half of all bipolar people have abused alcohol or drugs.

This can of course lead to heightened bipolar symptoms—and the many problematic behaviors that go along with them.

Also, despite the boastfulness that often accompanies mania, many untreated bipolar people prove unable to take care of themselves as independent adults. They often end up homeless, living in poverty, or under the guardianship of an uncaring person.

There also is the sheer waste of life. People with bipolar disorder might lose as many as nine years from their lives due to the general abuse to the body and mind that can accompany their condition. They can lose as many as twelve years of health, and fourteen years of productivity. Besides dealing with episodes, untreated bipolar people might also lose valuable time trying to put their lives back in order *after* a major episode.

 Fact

> The diminished capacity defense is used to argue that a defendant did not know right from wrong when harming another. As bipolar disorder becomes more commonly diagnosed, news headlines feature more stories of murders committed by a non-medicated bipolar person. Considerable controversy surrounds these cases: Did the perpetrator know right from wrong when he committed the crime?

How Loved Ones Are Affected

As the bipolar person spirals further out of control, others might mourn their sense of loss as though someone has died. In a sense, this can be true, as the child or young adult they used to know just does not seem to be there anymore. In other cases, the bipolar person has a fair amount of cogent moments. But because there is always the fear and dread that they may have another episode, others start to keep their distance anyway. And so once again, they end up missing the person they used to know.

Especially when the bipolar person is otherwise a creative and engaging person, there can be a real sense of loss. A young protégé might feel deeply pained having to sever ties with a mentor who could have helped him—but he just could not take the mentor's mood swings anymore.

Loss of Sleep, Time, and Energy

Some people find their lives to be virtually at the mercy of someone else's bipolar disorder. Getting awakened at odd hours, having to listen to someone or drive her someplace—or bail her out of jail—becomes a full-time job. Sometimes, people will end up canceling other social or professional plans in order to take care of the bipolar person's latest crisis.

When the mania switches to depression, it can also be time-consuming for others. Because they want the person to "snap out of it," they go out of their way to spend time with them, or run errands or do favors for them. If the depression seems serious enough, others can also spend a great deal of time simply worrying, or wondering what the problem is.

Loss of Money

There are many ways a bipolar person can cause a loved one to lose money. Maybe the bipolar person will simply take it, or invest it in a manically driven scheme that fails. Also, bipolar people might constantly borrow money, having spent or lost all of their own. Or, if they are unable to hold down a job, they might ask to borrow money because they need to eat or pay the rent.

In other instances, bipolar people might ask for financial assistance because of some sort of trouble they are in. Maybe they need to get bailed out of jail, pay a fine, or make restitution. If young and naïve, someone might get swept up in the bipolar person's manic frenzy, and likewise spend too much money in the name of having fun.

When bipolar people are depressed, others might spend money on them in order to cheer them up. Or maybe they just want to make sure the bipolar person is eating and attending to other basic needs.

However it happens, there is no guarantee that the bipolar person will pay the money back. Many people find that knowing a bipolar person is an expensive proposition.

Loss of Direction

If someone spends a great deal of their life caring for or worrying about a bipolar person, the result might be that they themselves accomplish very little. Their own goals and plans remain forever out of reach as they instead try to save or protect the individual with serious mood disorder. The next thing these caregivers know, months, years, or even decades have gone by, and they still are not calling their lives their own.

Not only are mental and physical energy sometimes misdirected, but people might also, for example, not go to college in order to care for the bipolar person. Sometimes, what should have been pleasant memories (weddings, vacations) get spoiled because of someone's untreated mental condition.

Furthermore, children of bipolar parents who are not receiving treatment are likely to be denied basic nurturing and socialization that help to ensure a successful life. Such children might grow up with very little sense of security about life, because from one moment to the next they never knew what their parent was going to be like.

 Question

Clearly, untreated bipolar disorder can have damaging emotional effects; but are there also negative physical effects?
One recent study has shown that untreated bipolar disorder causes serious brain damage over time. People who have been untreated for the longest amount of time are more likely to have lowered levels of the amino acid N-acetylaspartate in the right hippocampus of the brain. This leads to less effective functioning of neurons and axons, and hence diminished functioning.

When confronted with someone's mania, the loved one might be insulted, yelled at, belittled, laughed at, or bullied. When depression takes over, the loved one might feel guilty for not feeling as bad, or unworthy of happiness. Or maybe the depression is so intense, it seems to pervade everything.

Of course, sometimes the opposite happens: Someone becomes determined to prove that "sick" relative wrong, and becomes obsessed with success, or saving the world. It takes a rare spirit to avoid these pitfalls of extremes when growing up around untreated bipolar disorder.

Making everything that much sadder is that the bipolar individual might well be basically a good and kind person who does not mean to act out in these ways, but who literally cannot help it. On balance, much unhappiness is generated for all concerned when the bipolar person does not get treatment. However, sometimes the reasons for not getting treatment are complicated.

When Patients Accept Diagnosis, but Treatment Fails

As previously mentioned, treatment for bipolar has about a 60 percent success rate. But what about the other 40 percent? The fact is that some people are willing to accept a doctor's diagnosis that they are bipolar, but for one reason or another the treatment ends up not working.

Side Effects of Medication

About 20 percent of bipolar patients who seek treatment report or experience harmful side effects from medication. These side effects might be genuine, as when a doctor notices a dangerous change in blood-cell count, or when a patient honestly is experiencing (for example) severe nausea, or even just discomfort. In other instances, patients might be exaggerating the side effects, imagining them, or even lying outright about them.

But regardless of how or why, the effect is usually the same: the patient goes off the medication. There might be an effort made to find a substitute medication, which might succeed or fail. However, in some instances, patients might decide to not even try other treatments. They feel that the side effects were actually *worse* than enduring episodes of mania or depression. Having survived such episodes in the past, they decide they can survive them again in the future.

With all due respect for the discomfort—or even danger—of certain side effects, patients should continue to find a workable combination with their doctors. The alternative of living without any medication is likely to be the most dangerous possibility of all.

Finding the Right Combination

Bipolar disorder includes both mania and depression. There can also be other complications that signal a need for antipsychotic medication, sleep aids, or anti-anxiety pills. Unfortunately, sometimes one medication can react negatively with another, causing harmful side effects. Or one medication might more or less make another ineffective. In still other instances, an antidepressant, for example, can heighten mania. Or maybe a patient does not respond to one mood stabilizer, so another is tried . . . and this *new* one does not work well with the antidepressant.

If a patient is not wholly responding to a combination of medications—if many symptoms are under control, but not all of them are—the doctor must make a decision as to whether or not to let things be, or to keep trying. Hopefully, the wisest possible decision is made, though sometimes there are errors in judgment.

Additional Disorders

Some people are both bipolar and schizophrenic—or bipolar with Down syndrome, or with AD/HD, or some other mental disorder. In such instances, treatment becomes that much more complicated. The issue of finding the right combination of medications is even more challenging, and the likelihood of harmful side effects increases.

Moreover, if one doctor diagnoses (for example) bipolar with some schizophrenia, another doctor might decide there is only bipolar disorder present—or vice versa. And so the new doctor changes the medication regime, more tests and observations are needed, and an ultimate workable treatment lies that much farther in the future.

No Response to Medication/Misdiagnosis

Something like 20 percent of bipolar patients either do not respond to medication, or else stop responding to it after a while. An assortment of other medications can be tried out, but perhaps nothing seems to work for very long—or to work at all. Or maybe the mania is under control, but not the depression.

Some patients might keep on trying to find the right medication. But others might reach a point where they feel they have tried enough different kinds, and will simply make do as best they can without it. In some instances, doctors might prescribe alternate therapies such as electroshock therapy, but the patient—or his legal guardian—must agree to such a dramatic step.

 ## Fact

Ethnic minorities are more likely to be misdiagnosed when it comes to mental disorders. Reasons for this include disproportionately high rates of poverty (which limit access to adequate medical care), cultural and communication differences, and a tendency for some groups to mistrust doctors and instead rely on family or religious leaders to deal with these issues.

Particularly in the category of patients who do not respond to treatment, the possibility of misdiagnosis must also be considered. You may also recall the category of bipolar disorder not otherwise specified, or Bipolar NOS. The patient certainly *seems* bipolar, but some of the symptoms do not fit the usual categories. For example, based on what the patient says, it is hard to tell if he is Bipolar II or has cyclothymia. And Bipolar III emerges when a patient being treated for depression develops manic symptoms. The doctor must be able to correctly recognize that this is indeed a new development caused by the medication.

Also, sometimes patients themselves overdramatize their symptoms. Doctors are trained to recognize this, but some might not do so all of the time, and instead make a misdiagnosis.

Whatever the reason, both doctor and patient might continue to believe that bipolar disorder is present when such is not the case.

When Patients Accept Diagnosis, but Resist Treatment

Another possibility is that the patient believes the diagnosis of bipolar disorder, but refuses treatment for it. This pattern can take several basic forms, including never even trying medication, going off medication temporarily, or going off medication permanently.

Never Even Trying Medication

Some patients might be willing to accept that they are bipolar, but they do not even attempt to get proper treatment. Generally, it is difficult to force people to take medication unless they are committed to a medical facility, are under someone else's legal guardianship, or have otherwise been ordered by the court to do so.

Sometimes, people simply are too deeply enmeshed in their mood extremes to get treatment. The depression seems so pervasive that they do not think there is reason to hope. Or the mania is such that the person thinks nothing is wrong, it is just that everyone else has a problem.

In other cases, patients listen to someone other than a doctor. There might be a friend or family member who says that all medications are bad, or that they read about a celebrity who had a negative experience being on medication. Or maybe someone tells the patient that they know a religion, faith healer, or self-improvement group that can "cure" bipolar disorder. Sometimes, too, well-meaning (but misinformed) people will say that it is really just a matter of more Vitamin D, or going vegetarian, or more daily fiber or exercise. In any case, this other person is trusted more than the doctor, so the patient decides against following medical advice.

Another possibility is that the patient is afraid to go against the friend or family member. Rather than risk the anger or disapproval of this person, the patient sadly decides that living with untreated bipolar episodes is the lesser of two evils. Particularly if the patient has been unable to work and take care of himself, this other person or persons might have an extremely powerful influence.

L. Essential

Some bipolar people might simply decide within themselves not to get treatment. Besides media influences, some people might firmly believe that medication is always wrong—that instead they must learn to train their minds differently, or face something from their past. Such people often think that medication is an artificial and cowardly approach that does not work.

Like anyone else, bipolar people might have other kinds of issues they need to work on. And there is also evidence that certain traumas and bad lifestyle choices can help manifest inherent bipolar symptoms. But someone is *not* bipolar solely because they never got over their parents' divorce, or never had the confidence to seek the career of their dreams.

Going Off Medication Temporarily

One of the main reasons for a patient to temporarily stop treatment is the apparent absence of creativity when on medication. Some people who write, paint, compose, act, direct, sing, or dance are unable to find a way to harness their creative energy within the more mild range of moods that medication yields. Most commonly, patients state that they "miss" the mania—the high highs. While most creative bipolar people report that they can still do their craft under medication—or even do it better—there are about 20 percent who state that they cannot. Whether they are being honest or not, the outcome is the same: They go off medication for the day, week, or month that they will be giving a performance or finishing a project.

Medications must continue to be refined in ways that enable all patients to maintain their creative natures. But in the meantime, temporarily going off medication is problematic in several ways:

- **Once off of medication, many of the old thoughts and behaviors return.** So, the patient ends up not going back on medication after all. Episodes return, and the patient pays a very high price for finishing that novel or giving that concert. Perhaps real harm is done to the self or another.
- **Back within the throes of mania in particular, the patient might decide that no medication is needed ever again.** For example, the euphoric self-confidence is such that patients might decide that the only reason they were medicated was because other people were "jealous" of them. Or perhaps the patient flip-flops between taking medication and not, which makes it ineffective.
- **One might question the values of society.** "Success" would seem to be worth attaining at any cost to the self or loved ones. In effect, the message seems to be: "Sure, he was miserable and killed himself and made life hell for his family, but now his paintings are worth a lot of money." Acclaim seems to be more important to some than basic happiness.
- **Some famous creative people will tell reporters that they go off their medications from time to time to get the creative juices flowing and thereby send out a questionable message.** People who do not have the same support systems as celebrities might decide that if the famous and successful So-and-So can go off medication now and then, so can they.

Going Off Medication Permanently

Many of the reasons for permanently going off medication have to do with harmful side effects, or the medication not working, as previously discussed. Still other people might resent having to spend so much time getting their blood tested, answering questions, monitoring themselves, and so on. Sometimes these are people who lead extremely busy lives, and it is a challenge to make room for all these extra activities. In other instances, people might simply resent the hassle of proper treatment. For example, the doctor's office might be hard to get to, or the patient have a strong dislike for blood tests.

 # Fact

On February 7, 2001, an untreated bipolar patient named Robert Pickett fired several shots at the White House before getting wounded in the knee by Secret Service. Pickett was a former West Point cadet who was eventually fired by the IRS and claimed the government was persecuting him. President Bush was not at the White House at the time.

In other situations, patients might feel insulted by the doctor(s) or staff. If you do not fully grasp that bipolar disorder is an illness that you did not cause, you might feel shame about having it. And so if you think the medical community treats you "like a child," or "like a crazy person," your pride is deeply wounded. You might even decide that you do not need all these people and their silly, insulting medications, and that you can get better on your own.

There also are patients who continue to feel overwhelmed by the notion that bipolar disorder means keeping up treatment forever—always taking medication every day, and always returning to the doctor for check-ups. Some might decide that there *has to* be a better way of dealing with it on their own. However, once again, such efforts can only fail.

When Patients Resist Diagnosis and Treatment

Finally, there are people who not only refuse treatment, but they also refuse to believe that they are bipolar. This refusal to accept even the diagnosis of bipolar frequently is caused by denial. Unless symptoms have escalated to full-scale Bipolar I, it can be all too easy to rationalize them away. And even people having a major manic attack might be shrouded in denial. This can be self-denial, or the denial of others who insist that the problem is anything but bipolar disorder. Whether before or after a diagnosis has been made, denial is one of the most daunting obstacles to treatment and normality.

The tricky thing about these denial mechanisms is that sometimes they are true. Maybe the cause *is* something more minor than bipolar disorder. Or maybe both are true—the person is bipolar *and* doing this other thing. The problem is when bipolar disorder is automatically excluded as a possibility—when people are convinced the problem is only the minor excuse being offered.

 Alert

Denial on the part of family members and loved ones is especially high in the calm between the storm—the periods between episodes. It is then that the last episode can more easily be dismissed as a "bad dream" that like all dreams did not really happen. Maybe it was just something else the matter with the bipolar person—or maybe everyone else overreacted. For this reason, family therapy is often recommended for the bipolar patient.

In other instances, there is extreme ignorance or superstition surrounding the entire issue of mental illness. People think that they or their loved one cannot possibly be bipolar, because only "crazy" people are bipolar. And as "everyone" knows, these "crazy" people are demonic, sub-human, weak, bad, or any number of other stereotypes.

Some people also do not understand that bipolar disorder has a basis in brain chemistry—and so they think it reflects badly on themselves and/or their families. Not only do some people worry that a mentally ill loved one means that they were "bad" parents, but some mentally ill patients are unwilling to accept their diagnosis because they do not want to believe that they *had* bad parents.

In still other situations, there can be shame about the family bloodline. These people *do* believe that mental illness can be genetically transmitted; in fact, they believe this so strongly that they refuse to accept that anyone in their own bloodline could be mentally ill. This is a misplaced form of family pride that helps no one.

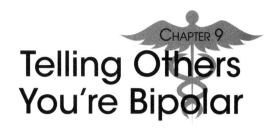

CHAPTER 9

Telling Others You're Bipolar

Telling other people about your diagnosis as bipolar is a very complex, personal decision. How do you know who to tell, and when? How much information should you give? What if you feel uncomfortable sharing the information at all? Do you treat the issue differently in your personal life than your professional life? These are just some of the issues likely to arise once a diagnosis has been made. This chapter offers advice on dealing with the situation.

Why Do You Want to Tell?

Before trying to figure out what to say to whom about having bipolar disorder, it is a good idea to be clear as to why you are telling a certain person—or anyone at all—about it. What do you hope to accomplish? Essentially, there are reasonable goals that can be achieved by sharing this information, as well as unreasonable goals.

Reasonable Goals

Reasonable goals are ones that are possible to achieve. This does not mean you will achieve them—sometimes, of course, things go wrong—but it is realistic to hope that these goals might be achieved:

- **Reveal the secret.** It probably bothers you that certain people do not know that you are bipolar. In this case, it can be a big relief to finally be up front about your situation. Telling others accomplishes your goal of making your secret burden a known reality.

- **Offer an explanation.** While there is no guarantee that others will accept what you say, you can at least try to explain some of your past behavior by talking about being bipolar. Discussing the matter openly can clear up aspects about you in the minds of others.

- **Apologize, if appropriate.** It's true that you cannot help being bipolar and so have not always had full control over things you've said and done. Nonetheless, when explaining about being bipolar, you might feel better if you offered an apology to certain people for past words or deeds. Of course, they may accept or reject your apology.

- **Answer some questions.** If people have questions about what bipolar means or how it relates to your situation, you can answer these questions to the best of your ability.

- **Offer other resources.** You can let people know about books or Web sites focused on bipolar disorder, as well as support services for loved ones.

Unreasonable Goals

Besides the previous reasonable goals, there also are some unreasonable goals that you might have when it comes to sharing about being bipolar. Before you get your heart set on achieving these unreasonable goals, remember the following points:

- **You cannot control others' reactions.** Some people might be accepting and supportive, while others might react with disbelief, anger, or shame. Some might be happy that you shared; others might cry. Some might stay an active part of your life, while others might decide to keep their distance. If you offer an apology, some people might accept it, and some might not.

- **You cannot predict who will be supportive.** You might be surprised by which people react with positive support, and which people are dismissive, or even angry. Sometimes people seem very "nice," but it is just a defensive front they put up because they cannot deal well with life's complications. And so these people might try to convince you that nothing is really the matter—or start ignoring you.

- **You cannot control how others will use the information.** Even when sworn to secrecy, sometimes people cannot resist sharing a secret with others. If you confide in certain people, you should not be too disappointed if it turns out that one or more has spread the word. Also, even if you say, for example, that you do not want to be treated any differently, some people might start to do so—especially if they have heard about your being bipolar as gossip from someone else.

- **You cannot predict how you will feel afterward.** Hopefully, you will feel relieved and cleansed for having shared. But it is possible that you will instead feel worried and upset. Maybe it does not go as well as you hoped. Or maybe it goes well on the surface, but you sense that underneath it all someone was very uncomfortable. If you are confiding in people simply to get a good feeling, you might be in for a disappointment. You may feel closer to some people for having shared, but you also might feel less close.

- **You cannot expect your symptoms to vanish once you tell.** Sometimes people think that by telling other people about a problem they have, it will somehow make the problem go away. Feel free to let your loved ones know what is going on with you, but do not expect it to do more than it does. Honesty is its own reward.

Achieving Honesty

Before you tell anyone else about being bipolar, it is good to be honest with yourself about it first. After all, you cannot expect someone else to understand something if you do not understand it yourself. This might seem an overwhelming task. But pretend for a moment that a movie is being made about your life as a bipolar person. Then think about how the story would unfold, scene by scene.

L. Essential

When explaining to someone about bipolar disorder, you might want to keep it as simple as possible. Even the most attentive listener's mind will start to wander after about five minutes. And some research indicates that on average people pay attention to one out of every ten points that a speaker makes.

First, what led up to your diagnosis? What were some of the experiences or thoughts that led you to seeing a doctor? Did you always feel different from other people? Did you try to pretend that nothing was wrong? Did you say or do things you regretted before being diagnosed?

Next, how did you feel when you were told? Was it a relief to know that there was a name for what had been troubling you? Or were you sad to find out—or afraid, or ashamed, or all three?

Third, what, if anything, is different now that you have started treatment? How do you feel about yourself now? Is the medication making a difference? What are some of the challenges you still are facing?

Fourth, where do you see yourself headed? In the movie of your life, what would you want to say at this time before "The End"? Would the movie end on a hopeful note? A sad note? Who do you see yourself as being right now?

Finally, in what ways are you the same person you always were? Finding out you are bipolar obviously changes many things. But it does not change everything. You still probably have many of the same personal interests, likes and dislikes, and care for the same people. As your medication has a stabilizing effect, think about what has *not* changed about the things you say and do—the things that matter to you, bipolar or not.

If you do not have much confidence in your ability to talk about bipolar disorder, or to talk about it to a particular person—or if in general you do not feel you communicate very well—there are several alternatives to consider:

- **Write it down.** Some people are better at writing down their thoughts than saying them face-to-face. Word processors make it especially easy to rewrite your ideas until you have them the way you want them. Even if it is your spouse, mother, child, or best friend, you can always write a letter rather than risk explaining something the wrong way.

- **Seek out additional materials.** If you know of a book, pamphlet, video, or Web site that you think will help you to say what you mean, feel free to use them. It is not "cheating" to rely on additional resources.

- **Ask loved ones to help.** If you already have one or more people who know you are bipolar and are highly supportive, don't be afraid to ask them to help you in explaining it to other people who you fear might be less supportive. It's probably a good idea to make sure that everyone already knows everyone else; it can be awkward to have strangers meeting for the first time over something so important.

- **Ask your doctor to help.** Your psychiatrist probably will not have the time to have dozens of special meetings with your loved ones. But if you would like to schedule, say, one or two special sessions in which the doctor is present to help explain what is going on, it can probably be arranged.

Telling People in Your Personal Life

Once you have figured out what you would like to say, a good way of saying it, and if you are clear about what your goals are for sharing, you will want to decide with whom to share it all. You should not automatically feel that you should tell everyone you encounter. It is perfectly normal to feel more comfortable sharing the information with some people and not others. First and foremost, you need to figure out who you will tell in your personal world—and what you might say.

 Alert

> When you tell your children that you're bipolar, be careful not to turn them into your caregivers; they should still be able to be kids. You might want to talk to your doctor to discuss your specific situation before deciding how to proceed. It is also reasonable to expect that there will be many questions and discussions with your children over time, especially if they are quite young. One of the most important points to make clear to your children is that they are not at all to blame for your condition.

Immediate Family

There are people in your immediate family who absolutely need to know about your diagnosis, while with others it is optional. For instance, a spouse obviously has every right to know that you are bipolar. If you are dating someone and it is getting at all serious, this person should be told. It is extremely unfair to enter into a committed relationship without sharing such important information. You might also decide to tell a former spouse, in order to make peace with your past. However, you should check with a lawyer first, if there is a possibility that the former spouse could use this information against you.

Your children also have a right to know you are bipolar. Especially if they are grown—and even if your relationship is strained—they should be told. As for younger children still living at home, there is no magic age by which they are old enough to handle the information. Some children are more mature than others. You should also assume that children are even less likely than adults to keep a secret. If you tell one of your children, but not the other, you are putting both children in an awkward position.

As for your parents: besides simply wanting to confide in them, you might want to share your diagnosis if you think it might also apply to another family member. If you have difficulty communicating with one or more parent, you will want to take extra care in planning out what to say. But assuming both parents are living, try to avoid telling one parent, but not the other. Remember, couples—sometimes even ex-couples—confide in each other, especially in matters pertaining to their children. Or one parent might use this information to show how much closer you are to her or him. So you might be setting yourself up for a complicated "he said/she said" situation if you tell one parent but not the other.

Some parents blame themselves if their children have mental issues—or else assume that other people will. Without meaning to hurt you, a parent might say something extremely disconfirming. Before disclosing to your parents about being bipolar, you should consider how responsive they have tended to be over the years. Have they encouraged you to seek professional help, or did they act as if nothing was wrong? Your task will be much more difficult when there has been denial. If you feel you should tell them anyway, you should make it clear that your purpose is not to blame them. You also might especially consider getting help from your doctor or other sources before talking to them.

Siblings also might be told. Unless a brother or sister has direct control over your finances or career, you probably do not have much to lose by sharing about being bipolar. Different siblings are of course close or not close, but when it comes to something this serious many will be supportive even if they normally are not. Some might say they do not think the diagnosis is right, or that they do not believe in medication for mood disorders. But if you are your own adult, in the final analysis this opinion probably will not stop you from doing what you need to do with your life.

Others in Your Personal Life

Like anyone else, the people in your personal life are blood relatives (whom you did not get to choose) and your spouse and/or close friends (whom you probably *do* get to choose). Bipolar or not, hopefully the people you *choose* to have in your life are worthy of your trust. As for extended relatives, you might need to decide on a case-by-case basis. In any event, you might feel like you want some friends or extended relatives to know more than others.

When it comes to extended relatives, it probably will be less traumatic to tell your grandparents, cousins, aunts, uncles, and step-relatives about being bipolar. If you have an unusually close relationship with any of them—if a grandmother or uncle is like a parent to you—then treat that person accordingly. If you have a volatile relationship with any of these extended relatives, you might prefer they not know.

 Fact

Studies indicate that most adults are likeliest to confide important information to their spouses, followed by their best friends. Parents are less likely to be confided in by adults. If as an adult you seldom confide in your parents, you are not alone. But if it is difficult for you to confide in your spouse, you need to seriously reconsider your relationship.

Some families congregate more than others. If, for example, your parents frequently see your cousins, aunts, and uncles, it might be unrealistic to assume that this information will be kept from these other relatives indefinitely. Your parents have their own lifetime of experience with these people, and might want to confide in them.

So unless you strongly do not want any of these other relatives to know about it, you might want to tell them yourself.

On the other hand, if you seldom if ever see these other kinds of relatives, there is probably no pressing need to tell them. In fact, if you do, they might even resent knowing, and feel it was none of their business.

Since you choose your friends, they should be people that you feel you can confide in. Otherwise, they probably are not much of a friend. If a so-called friend wants nothing more to do with you after you share about being bipolar, you probably have not lost much.

Some well-meaning friends might try to "help" by saying you could not really be bipolar, or that you should not be taking medication to treat it. But again, if they are truly your friends, they will respect your decision as an adult to get the help you need.

Besides telling friends about your diagnosis, you should also let them know how much you do or do not want to talk about it. Probably it is a good idea to answer their initial questions, but if they keep bringing it up more than you want to keep talking about it, you should say so—in a nice way.

Telling People in Your Professional Life

Though revealing that you're bipolar may be a given when it comes to close family and friends, telling people you work with can bring up entirely separate and possibly more complex issues. This complexity is only enhanced if your job includes being in the public eye.

Bosses and Coworkers

There are several reasons why it might be a good idea to tell people at work that you're bipolar. One obvious reason would be that you are close friends with someone. If a coworker or boss is someone with whom you socialize outside the office, and you have successfully confided in this person in the past, you can probably trust her. Moreover, the person might feel insulted if she ends up hearing the information from someone else.

You also might need special arrangements made for your situation. For example, if you must take an extra-long lunch hour every Wednesday to see your doctor, you will want to inform your employer. Unless your work performance is otherwise problematic, or unless there is a legal pre-existing policy in place given the nature of the work, it is illegal to fire you simply because you are disclosing your diagnosis.

There also can be other legal considerations. You might want to consult an attorney first, but some professions might require disclosure of information such as being diagnosed with a mood disorder. If you or other people might be put at risk because, for example, one of your medications makes you drowsy, it might be best for all concerned to bring the matter up before something unfortunate happens.

⌇ Essential

Self-disclosure is the act of sharing something about yourself that the other person probably did not know. One of the hidden expectations of self-disclosure is that the other person will likewise share a secret about himself. This is called the norm of reciprocity.

You also might wish to foster a general atmosphere of trust. You might be in a professional situation in which you know absolutely that no one can or would use your diagnosis against you. If you feel like you want to educate people on bipolar disorder, or simply would feel good about sharing who you are, you might well have nothing to lose by doing so.

Your Public Life

Separate from your professional life is your public life. Celebrities of course have an active public life. But even if you are not a famous person, it is possible to go public with being bipolar. For example, you could be the subject of a local news story, or speak in public forums about being someone with a mood disorder. In other words, you can come completely out of the closet about being bipolar, and anyone who meets you in the future might know you as that person who was on the evening news as having bipolar disorder.

This can be a useful step for you and for raising public awareness. However, you should not feel that you *have to* do this. Here are some questions to consider:

- **Are you a private person?** This might seem an obvious point, but it is important. Before being diagnosed bipolar, did you mind much, for example, if people knew you were divorced, or flunked a French class, or were bisexual, or had a nose job, or anything else about you that could have been kept more private? If you are sensitive when it comes to being criticized or gossiped about, going public might be more than you can handle.

- **Are you a good speaker?** Are you someone who is praised for being articulate, or do you often feel that you could have said something better? You do not want to say anything in public that might make you appear foolish. You also do not want to say anything that could get twisted around by a reporter, or taken out of context. Previous experience with public speaking or dealing with the media is helpful. Short of this, you could read a book, take a class, or get advice from others as to how to best present yourself.

- **Does your story educate, inspire, or motivate?** There are three good reasons for going public about being bipolar. You can seek to educate people as to what bipolar disorder is, and how it is treated. You can also strive to inspire people with your story, to give hope to other people who are bipolar or who have a loved one that is. A third reason is to motivate people to take action. For example, perhaps you would like to see more government support for research.

If your answer to all three of these questions is no, then you might want to think again about why you want to go public. Disclosing to the general public about anything personal can sometimes have a strong emotional effect on the person who is disclosing. You want to make sure that you are not doing something that might make you vulnerable to either the inflated grandiosity that can come with mania, or the feeling of worthlessness that can come from depression.

Fielding Questions

When you share about being bipolar, there are many kinds of questions you might be asked in response. Some might be technical questions about the nature of the disorder. Other questions might be about you. By all means answer anything you feel confident about answering; but also remember that it is all right to say, "I don't know." When it is the truth—when you really do not know the answer—then this is actually a wise statement. Only foolish people pretend to know something when they do not. No one knows everything all the time.

Technical Questions

If someone asks you something about bipolar disorder and brain chemicals, or about genetics, and it is beyond your level of understanding, by all means say so. The same holds true if you are asked, for example, how your hypomania differs from cyclothymia, and you do not honestly know the answer. Sophisticated questions about how your medication works, or how it differs from other medication, might likewise be answered with "I don't know," if such is indeed the case.

Especially when the person you are talking to might in the future need to have accurate information as to the nature of bipolar disorder, it is important that you do not make anything up. Furthermore, if your manic phases rendered you unable to admit to being wrong about anything, it could be an important exercise in trust building to freely admit to not having all the answers.

However, what you can do is suggest a source that might provide the answer. You can offer to ask your doctor the same question. If you have access to a computer, perhaps the two of you could look the information up on the Internet—or go to a library and read a book together. If you have to give the answer "I don't know" frequently, it's a strong sign that you need to become more educated about your condition.

Questions about Your Past

You might be asked if something you said or did in the past was a symptom of being bipolar. Sometimes it might be easy to answer yes or no, because you do have a clear sense of when you were having an episode. But if you are not sure, you should be honest and say so. Obviously, people do get angry or depressed or arrogant—or make foolish, impulsive decisions—without necessarily having a bipolar episode. So if the situation was ambiguous, it is okay to not be sure why you did what you did.

Once again, honesty is important here. After all, the point in discussing your bipolar disorder is for people to understand you better, so there is little point in giving an answer that might be misleading, just for the sake of giving an answer. And still again, it might be important for other reasons to have your loved ones get accurate answers, in case they witness a future episode.

Questions about Your Future

Still other questions might concern what you plan to do from here: Will you keep working—or start looking for work, as the case may be? What if you develop serious side effects from the medication? Will you be able to go on long vacations away from your doctor? Are you going to contact your former spouse? The list of possible questions is virtually endless.

You might well have a sense of how you plan to handle certain matters in the future. But, again, if you do not know what you will be doing about something, say so. You should not make promises you cannot keep, nor should you give people false hopes. You also want to avoid creating avoidable conflicts over promising more than you can deliver.

Additionally, for your own well-being, you do not want to take on more than you reasonably can. If you already have a history of losing jobs, flunking classes, losing money, or getting divorced, you do not need to continue adding blemishes to your record. So do not over-commit yourself just because you're afraid of disappointing someone. Instead, try to work out with your doctor what is a reasonable goal that you can obtain. And you can say as much to other people—that you will ask your doctor if he or she thinks this is something you can handle.

 Fact

Many bipolar people find they have trouble holding down a job. Research indicates that bipolar disorder makes the likelihood of someone being employed 40 percent less likely. However, at the same time, higher levels of lithium are significantly associated with improved work performance.

You Don't Have to Tell Everyone

When all is said and done, there are perfectly valid reasons for wanting to share the fact that you are bipolar with other people. But there can also be perfectly valid reasons for not sharing this information—or at least not yet.

Is Your Medication Working?

If your medication has not yet started to work, or if you are having problems finding the right combination of medications, you might decide to wait before talking to other people about it. Maybe you feel it is appropriate to go ahead and share, but if you think there are people whom you would be worrying more than you have to, you might decide to wait at least a short while. You might feel that all concerned are better off with your being able to say: "Not to worry, my treatment is working." Particularly if your loved one is very young or very old, you might decide to wait.

Timing

If something else major is going on in your life, you might want to wait until it is over to share your bipolar news. This major thing might be good news—your cousin is getting married in a week—or sad news, such as an old friend just passed away.

But being bipolar is big news in itself, and it deserves proper attention. It should not be talked about for the first time while everyone is in the middle of planning a wedding—or a funeral, or some other major event.

Your Personal Comfort Zone

Besides there being good reasons for putting off telling certain people, you might also decide that there are some people you would just as soon *never* know about it. If, for example, you and a sibling just do not get along and she lives far away, you should not feel as though you *have to* tell her that you are bipolar.

Your own needs figure into things. There is such a thing as reasonably challenging yourself, but there is also such a thing as pushing yourself too far. If someone has always made you feel unsafe, you should not feel absolutely obligated to tell him something so personal about yourself.

CHAPTER 10

Lifestyle Choices

Medications such as mood stabilizers and antidepressants are essential in the treatment of bipolar disorder. Once episodes are minimized, the bipolar individual can make wise lifestyle choices. Then there can be less of a chance that a crisis will emerge that triggers an episode, or compels someone to go off medication. These wise lifestyle choices are not so very different from those that non-bipolar people might also elect to make. But for bipolar people they can have a special meaning.

Finding the Right Job

A positive work situation makes an enormous difference in anyone's life. For a person with bipolar disorder, it can also mean helping to minimize the possibility of extreme shifts of mood. If you are bipolar and your job tends to "drive you crazy," it might be worthwhile to consider making a change.

Doing What Makes You Happy

An *occupation* is what you do for a living, while a *vocation* is what you feel is your true calling in life. Some people are fortunate enough to make a living off of their vocation—they pay the bills by doing what they feel they should be doing with their lives. Other people are fortunate in a different way. Their occupation is *not* their vocation, but they have made peace with this reality, and they do not suffer from things like substance abuse or profound unhappiness.

Then there are less fortunate people. Some of them do *not* make peace with the knowledge that what they do for a living is not what they really want to be doing. These people might well be profoundly unhappy and turn to things like substance abuse for solace.

Still other people suffer from an ironic situation. They do make a living at what they do best, but there are unintended side effects that make them unhappy. For example, someone can be a brilliant lawyer, but get so swept up in winning every case that he or she suffers a stroke or a nervous breakdown. Their occupation is their vocation—but it is leading them to unhappiness, maybe even an early death.

L. Essential

> Wisdom and honesty are needed to determine if you are doing what you really want to be doing with your life—and if doing this makes you feel happy and content, or if it makes you feel anxious and crazed. Sometimes people might be better off doing their second- or third-favorite thing for a living, because they will not have to suffer the intensity of such extreme moods.

As a bipolar person, even more than other people you need to determine what makes you *happy*. Not what you think you "should" do, or what will please or disappoint other people—or what pays the most. It does not have to be what you have always done, or always assumed you would do. Maybe the answer is to do what has always been your most cherished dream. But if going after that dream causes your life to fall apart in other ways, it might not be worth it. You might need to find a new dream.

Avoiding Vicious Cycles

The media is full of stories about celebrities who go into rehab, only to fall back into the same destructive cycles regarding substance abuse or diet once they start making movies or music again. Similar things happen every day to the average person. Some jobs for some people set in motion a vicious cycle of negative behaviors. It might be the occupation itself, or it might be the specific place the person works. Here are some questions to ask yourself about a job:

- Do you engage in substance abuse because of upsetting things that happen at work?
- Did you start smoking after taking on this job?
- Have your eating or sleeping patterns deteriorated since taking on this job?
- Do you regularly wake up in the middle of the night with anxiety over your job?
- Are you unable to enjoy your time away from work because you cannot stop thinking about it?
- Does your job fill you with anger and rage?
- Do you find yourself wishing that bad things would happen to the people you work with?
- Does the thought of returning to work make you depressed?
- Do you have much less of a social life since taking on this job?
- On your time off, do you want to stay in bed and hide from the world, or else engage in reckless behavior such as binge spending or compulsive sex?

If you have answered yes to even one of these items, you might want to consider making some kind of career change. It might mean switching careers, or it might mean simply finding a different position in the same field. Changing jobs takes a lot of effort, but it might be well worth it.

What If You Feel You Cannot Work?

Many bipolar people do not work. Some bipolar people find that they simply are not able to work very much. There are those who do not seem to find the right combination of medications, or who do not take medication, and so are unable to work full-time, or perhaps are unable to work at all. If you find yourself in one of these situations, there is no shame in admitting your limitations. If there is an alternative strategy for how you can maintain food, shelter, and other basic necessities, you owe it both to yourself and to others to make the wise choice.

 Alert

> The workplace may well contribute not only to stress, but to early death. Men on average do not live as long as women, and there is no biological explanation for this. Instead, it appears that men pay a price for having more of the jobs, and more of the higher status ones. The pressure of keeping these positions drives many men to poor health practices, stress, and early death.

This does not mean you have to permanently give up. You can still make yourself useful in other ways, helping out around the house or doing volunteer work for a worthy cause as you are able. You can also continue to see your doctor and keep trying to find a treatment that works more effectively. However, you should avoid putting yourself in a position where you are forced to live in abject poverty—or perhaps even become homeless. If some kind of work is needed to nominally meet your basic needs, keep trying to find a job that is within your comfort zone. Seek help from employment agencies if need be. Explain your situation, and perhaps something doable will come along.

An alternative to not working at all is trying to find some completely different line of work from what you have tried to do before. In today's world, most people have more than one career throughout their life course. You are hardly alone if you find yourself switching to a different line of work. It also is quite common for people to return to school to learn a different skill or field. Older, returning students (called "non-traditional students") are commonplace in today's colleges and universities. So there is no good reason to fear starting out in a new direction.

Essential

> If need be, you might consider applying for Social Security Disability Insurance (SSDI) or Supplemental Security Income (SSI). To find out about eligibility and how to apply, go to *www.ssa.gov*. Alternatively, you can contact your local Social Security Office.

Some people like to cling to old habits, even bad ones, simply because they are familiar. So some people might be afraid to let go of their job, because they have been at it for a long time and have actually gotten used to feeling unhappy all day. Others might claim to miss the rush of adrenaline as they proceed to do without food or sleep and to argue all day with the boss—or whatever dysfunctional permutation the job takes on. For a bipolar person, this can mean increasing the odds that there will be extreme shifts of mood.

Fact

> The Office of Disability of the Department of Labor offers recommendations for accommodating a bipolar worker. These can include ways of maintaining stamina, such as flexible or part-time work loads; and ways of maintaining concentration, such as frequent small breaks, small tasks, and a work environment with few distractions. To learn more, go to *www.dol.gov/odep/welcome.html*.

People to Avoid

Before going into treatment, a bipolar person might well have alienated a great many loved ones. Some formerly close friends might have completely distanced themselves, while others might be technically present but emotionally closed off. But even when bipolar people never lose the support of kind, loving people, they might well have attracted their fair share of negative influences. As the old saying goes, misery loves company, and someone who is behaving erratically is likely to attract other erratic people.

Those Who Interfere with Treatment

A bipolar person is wise to avoid various kinds of people, as they might try to discourage you from sticking to your treatment. Here is a general list of those to be wary of:

- **People with drinking or substance abuse problems who are not taking recovery measures:** If someone has several years of sobriety, she might well make a wise and positive friend. But if someone is actively using, she should be avoided. Misery loves company, and such a person's denial about needing help might be expressed in terms of trying to discourage you from taking your medication.
- **People with other addictions or compulsive behaviors who are not taking recovery measures:** Once again, people in recovery might be good to know, while people who are not in recovery might encourage you to join in their compulsions.
- **People with mood disorders who are not seeking help or taking medication:** Some mood disorders are treated with medication, some by therapy, and some by both. If it is apparent that this person has bipolar disorder, AD/HD, BPD, or some other mood disorder, and is not getting the proper help for it, it is best that this person be avoided.
- **People who try to convince the bipolar person to go off medication:** Whether it is because of religion, shame, or some other reason for wanting to control the bipolar person,

anyone who nags about how the bipolar person should stop taking medication is likely to be a negative influence.

- **People with serious eating issues who are not taking recovery measures:** Once again, if someone is recovering from conditions such as anorexia or bulimia, they can make a good friend. But anyone actively in the throes of these disorders can encourage bad habits in the bipolar person. The same would hold true for compulsive binge eaters who suffer from extreme obesity.

General Negative Influences

There are other kinds of people who are likely to be a negative influence. They do not necessarily know or care you are bipolar, but their general lifestyle could compel you to engage in behaviors that lead to mood swings. Watch out for the following personalities:

- **People who seldom sleep or slow down:** If someone is always on the go and never lets up, he is likely to be a negative influence on the bipolar person, encouraging behaviors associated with mania.
- **People who engage in criminal activities:** Obviously, anyone is wise to avoid involvement with a criminal. But bipolar people can be especially taken advantage of, and end up in highly volatile, even dangerous, situations.
- **People who engage in risky behavior:** People who spend a lot of money, lose a lot of money in bad investments, or put themselves in dangerous situations should likewise be avoided.
- **People who are excessive gossips:** Probably everyone gossips sometimes. But someone who seems to get a powerful rush by relentlessly talking about others behind their back—and probably in very critical terms—is not good to be around. This type of person can encourage numerous traits associated with manic grandiosity.

- **People who do not seem to like the bipolar person:** This might seem an obvious point. But some people might merely tolerate a bipolar person out of pity, or perhaps to feel superior, or because he or she does not have a lot of other friends. If someone is always being critical, especially about aspects associated with bipolar disorder, he or she is probably not a real friend, and is best avoided.

People to Seek Out

Fortunately, there are at least as many people worth getting to know as to avoid. These are people who will either have a positive effect on you as a bipolar person, or will have no particular effect one way or the other, and will treat you just like anyone else.

The following kinds of people are likely to be either benign or even positive influences in your life:

- **Bipolar people getting treatment:** Whether it be in a formal support group, or informally, you can benefit by knowing other bipolar people. You can encourage and understand each other in ways that no one else can. Also, you can offer each other helpful suggestions based on your experience.
- **People getting treatment for other mood disorders or other problems:** You also might find sympathetic souls in people who actively deal with their own mental or emotional issues. You can support and learn from each other. However, you should make sure that the treatment, therapy, or recovery program is for real—and that the person has been doing it for some time.
- **Sympathetic family members with knowledge of bipolar disorder:** Most everyone wants to feel connected to their roots. And when relatives understand what bipolar is and is not, they can make good confidants, helpers, or assistants. You probably do not want pity, but constructive help can be a

good thing. However, you should not take people's assistance for granted and should make an effort to return their favors.

ᒪ Essential

For all the talk about how different men and women are, both sexes rate a sense of humor, intelligence, and good listening skills as among the most important qualities they seek in companionship from others. These qualities in friends can be especially valuable to a bipolar person struggling to get her life back on track.

There also are people who can simply be good fun to know, and who carry a minimum of excess baggage. Seek out the following kinds of people to have as friends:

- **People with balanced lives:** If you meet someone who eats three square meals a day, gets a good night's sleep, fulfills her daily responsibilities, makes time for leisure activities, is neither a tightwad nor a spendthrift, and is neither a prude nor a sex addict, this just might be a good person to know.
- **People who treat you like an equal:** Someone who does not want to "fix" you out of pity, but who instead simply wants friendship or love, is likely to be worth knowing.
- **People whose company is enjoyable:** It is important for bipolar people to try to keep anger, gossip, and grandiosity to a minimum. If seeing someone makes you riled up with rage or feelings of superiority, it might be best to stop socializing with this person. You cannot change another person, so let that person be and instead find people whom you find attractive and worthwhile.
- **People who solve their problems:** Some people complain a lot, but they do not actually want anything to get better. Even when people offer solutions to their problems, they do not

act on them—they would rather keep complaining and making excuses for themselves. Healthy people work on fixing problems and moving on. These are people that can be fun to know, because they will not overly burden you with their woes.

Clearing Out Chaos

Coming home to mess and clutter can put even a happy person into a foul frame of mind. No one wants to do a task if she knows it is going to take an hour of digging through mess just to locate the needed object or information. If having a nice home sounds like an impossibly complicated task, read the following suggestions for how to make it doable.

Evaluate Your Environment

At a basic level, you can think of your home in terms of being orderly or chaotic. A chaotic home can fuel manic or depressive tendencies in most anyone. Here are some examples:

- Before leaving for work, you are frantically rushing around at the last minute because you cannot find your car keys in the mess of your house. Hence, your day gets off to a hyper, distracted start. You carry dread inside you over whether or not you will find your keys the next day.
- After a hard day at work, you come home to the same mess. This can make you feel even worse. Without even consciously realizing it, it can reinforce the notion that your life is a mess, or that life itself is ugly.
- Everyday tasks that no one enjoys but that have to get done can take twice as long, because you have to clear off space, or find what it is you are looking for. And so the task can be even more unpleasant. You might even put it off until the last minute—which can fill you with dread and gloom, and then make you hyper as you scramble to get it done.

- You are too embarrassed to have people come into your home because it looks so bad, or else people do not like coming over. This keeps you feeling somewhat secretive, and disconnected from other people. It also can reinforce a sense of inadequacy—"normal" people can have houseguests, but you cannot.
- Living in mess reinforces notions of unworthiness, and keeps you from feeling relaxed even in your own home. Thus, you are less likely to do nice things for yourself around the house—simple things such as taking a long, soothing bath, or having a nice dinner.
- Because it is so unpleasant to be home, you become overly restless and impatient to get out of the house. You stay out later than you should, spend too much money, or maybe even have sex with a stranger, just to avoid being home.

What Is an Orderly Home?

In contrast to the chaos described previously, consider the following scenarios:

- You open your eyes in the morning to pleasant surroundings. You do not fret about your car keys, because you have a place to keep them. You leave for work after a nice breakfast, feeling energized to face your day.
- Additionally, you enjoy coming home from work, because you like the home that you enter. You may or may not have much money, but there are at least a few objects in your home that you enjoy looking at and make you feel happy or inspired.
- It is time to pay the monthly bills, and so you turn on your favorite music and go to the drawer where you keep your checkbook, calculator, stamps, and envelopes. (Or if you pay your bills online, or have an online bill-paying service, you check the numbers.) A screw on a kitchen drawer needs tightening, but it only takes a moment to get the screwdriver

out of the toolbox, and fix it. The rest of the evening is yours to enjoy.

- You look forward to having friends come over. People often comment that they enjoy your home. You visit their homes, in return, and have active, normal friendships.
- Especially after a trying day at work, you enjoy making yourself a soothing hot bath. To be extra good to yourself, maybe you light a few candles around the tub. Or you treat yourself to a new DVD, or a new glass bowl for the living room that you've saved up to buy. You understand the importance of being good to yourself.
- Your home is your refuge; it truly does make you feel at home. At the same time, it is not a cocoon that hides you from the world, because you enjoy sharing it with other people.

It sounds easy to do, but it is important to *keep* it easy, and not take things too far.

 Fact

When it comes to perceiving everyday reality, most people are about 80 percent visual. People see much more than we hear, taste, smell, or touch. Thus, that which is visually pleasant versus unpleasant can make a major impact on how "reality" is perceived, whether you are bipolar or not.

Replace Fanaticism with Tranquility

Some people become so fanatical about neatness that they make life hell for others—or themselves. It is as if a home is not for living in, but just to be admired by others. These people often come across as domineering, yet underneath it all they often have very little sense of self, because they live to please other people. This type of fanaticism can suggest manic-like symptoms. It also can swing over to depression when, for example, the slightest thing in the house seems to be amiss.

Are You a Fanatic Around the House?

Ask yourself the following questions to get an idea of whether or not you're a fanatic around the house:

- Do you spend all your money, bounce checks, or run up huge credit cards bills in order to buy things for your home?
- Are you sometimes late for appointments or missing out on activities because you "must" clean around the house?
- Do you get more angry than necessary when someone disturbs something in your home?
- Are even the nice little things you do for yourself overly regimented? For example, do you decide you must take your evening bath at 7:30 P.M. and become extremely upset when a phone call compels you to take it instead at 8:00?
- Have people ever inquired as to whether you might be obsessive-compulsive?

If you answered yes to any of these questions, you have a problem to work on. Perhaps your house is a cluttered, unorganized mess, which leads you to obsess over it and the time you spend there. In this case, you need to take steps to improve the situation. If you come up with an organizational plan, it will be easier to keep things neat, as all items will have their proper place. If your house is already neat and organized but you still find yourself obsessing, then it is your own behavior that must be neatened up.

Ask for Help

A great way to be both relaxed and organized is to seek help from others. If you do not have much money, you can turn to the people you know. For example, you can invite people over to a painting party. Or simply ask family and friends to help you organize your place, or to go shopping with you—being careful, of course, not to overspend. Some people enjoy helping with these kinds of tasks, so do not be shy about asking.

If you do have some money to spare, by all means hire professionals. There are all sorts of house painters, carpenters, electricians, and handypersons listed in the phone book. You can also hire an interior designer, explaining your needs for a given room.

There also are professional organizers—people who design, build, or buy the shelves, closet organizers, file cabinets, or drawers that you need. These organizers will also work with you to develop easy ways of keeping things orderly and neat. They specialize in helping people who are sloppy around the house, so you should not feel embarrassed about not knowing how to do it by yourself.

L. Essential

If you have very poor housekeeping skills, you might consider contacting a housecleaning service in your area. Perhaps you can hire someone to come in once a week—or even once a month—to thoroughly clean up at a reasonable rate. If you cannot afford to pay someone to come in, maybe you can trade favors with a neighbor or friend: if she cleans your house once a week or twice a month, you will mow her lawn or walk her dog.

Through banks and online services, you can arrange to have your monthly bills automatically paid each month. If you simply do not trust online services—or computers—you might be able to hire an accountant to take care of your monthly expenses. You should ask for references, to make sure it is a reputable and honest service. (As a precaution, sign all the checks yourself once the accountant has prepared them.) Once again, if you cannot afford an accountant, you still might have a friend or relative who can do this for you, in exchange for your doing something for them.

CHAPTER 11

Getting in Touch with Yourself

There are still other steps you can take to stabilize your life. These efforts involve getting in touch with your inner and outer self, and also understanding more about how you relate to other people, and what to expect—or not expect—from them. You should also make an effort to be more keenly aware of the past, present, and future. With common sense and a strong support network, you should be able to take these kinds of steps toward a full and rewarding life.

Dealing with the Past

When you start getting treatment, another thing to think about is the impression you have made up to this point. There probably have been some instances in the past in which you said or did things beyond your control. Your past might well have an impact on how people relate to the present news that you're bipolar.

Some People May Be Relieved

Some people who have known you a while might well have figured out that something had to be the matter. And since these other people also have access to books, TV, and the Internet, they may have even made an educated guess that you have some sort of mood disorder. Perhaps some even encouraged you to seek professional help. But they did at least have a sense that *something* needed fixing. These are the people that are likeliest to say they are relieved that you finally got the help you needed, and that your problem turned out to have a name. They will probably be extremely supportive.

However, some might have already distanced themselves from you for their own safety, or other needs. It is important that you respect these boundaries. If, over time, you are able to build a more actively close relationship, that will be great. But you need to demonstrate that you can respect other people's needs. If properly medicated, this should be doable, especially if you are willing to change old behavioral patterns.

Some People May Refuse to Accept It

Other people who have known you a long time might have tried to ignore your erratic tendencies and to convince themselves that nothing was wrong. Maybe they were too self-involved to face the possibility that someone in their lives required serious attention, maybe they felt shame, or maybe they had difficulty accepting that anyone could actually have a mental condition that could not be controlled. Perhaps treating mental illness with medication is against their religion or belief system. Still another possibility is that they did not want to consider that they themselves might have mental issues.

Essential

Some recent research indicates that bipolar patients have an enlarged hippocampus on the left side (the rational side) of the brain. The hippocampus is where memories are stored. Contrastingly, patients with schizophrenia have a smaller hippocampus. The full implications of this apparent discovery are still being explored.

Whatever the reason, these people are likely to respond with denial—perhaps infused with anger. Still, underneath all the denial or anger, these people will probably not be that surprised. Defensive, maybe, but not surprised. Over time, they might concede that maybe, just maybe, your doctor was right after all. In the meantime, try to remember that it actually is not about you, but about something in themselves that they do not want to face.

Some People May Feel It's Too Little Too Late

If, in the throes of mania or depression, you said or did things that hurt or frightened others, there might be people who are unwilling to give you much of a chance. Medication or no medication, you might have wounded them too deeply for them to want you in their lives.

If you feel it is important to explain yourself to these people—or even to apologize—then do it for yourself. But you should not expect or demand that they completely forgive you. It is especially important that you do not come across as minimizing what you did. True, you could not control it, and you will gain nothing by endlessly blaming yourself or feeling guilty. But at the same time, another person's sense of well-being is not a trivial matter, and you should not treat it as such. Everyone has limits, and everyone has the right to set their own boundaries. Especially if you are divorced or estranged from the person, you should not try to push your way back in.

Some of these people will probably thank you for sharing, and then make it clear that they need to be somewhere else—that they appreciate that you have explained yourself, but that's about as far as things will go. Others might respond with anger, and feel you are just trying to make excuses for yourself. In these situations, it is probably best not to argue. Either cut the meeting short, or politely leave after letting the person vent a little while.

Dealing with Family Shame

Despite all that is known about mental illness, there are still people who think it is a curse or a sign of being a bad person. Upon hearing that a loved one is bipolar, these people might misguidedly decide that the most important thing is protecting the family "name." Rather than making sure the person gets the help needed, they might even try to dissuade the person from doing anything about it. Even if they support treatment, they might be horrified to learn that the person has shared with others about being bipolar, perhaps even going public. Family shame can be dealt with in a few social areas.

Religion

Some families belong to religious groups that disapprove of medication for mental disorders under any circumstance. According to these groups, it is always a mistake to get medication, and practicing the principles of the religion is the only way to heal or cure the person. Some of these groups might think the medical community is simply misguided. Others might think it is evil, abusive, or even satanic.

Parents who belong to these groups might outright forbid the child to be medicated. Adult family members are of course technically free to make their own choices, but sometimes they decide not to get treatment rather than present the family in a "negative" light. The results of such a decision are often tragic.

As previously discussed, if you are bipolar and religion is important to you, you might try to find a group that does not make such blanket judgments about treatment. Many religions have an alternate view that humankind should use its knowledge to help and heal.

Status or Class

Rich or poor, there are families who are extremely concerned with what other people think of them. They worry that if everything is not "perfect," others will judge them as unworthy. There is nothing wrong with wanting your loved ones to be successful, but some people are show-offs who cannot stop bragging about all their children or siblings are accomplishing. In such a family, it is possible that someone having bipolar disorder will be seen as lowering the family's status or class—as if only "inferior" families produce members with mood disorders.

In such instances, it might be helpful to point out the famous, distinguished people who have been likewise afflicted, and how bipolar disorder has often been associated with creativity. You also might teach your family that bipolar disorder is about brain processes, and not about being rich or poor.

Public position

Still other families might worry that because they are in the public eye, they cannot let it be known that a member of their clan has a mood disorder. They might even tolerate being blackmailed rather than have the "shameful" news go public. Perhaps the family is deeply enmeshed in politics or religion and worried that the public will distrust them if it learns that there is mood disorder within their ranks.

 Fact

> Notorious spree killer Charles Starkweather was executed at age nineteen in 1959. At one point, his attorneys urged him to plead insanity in order to spare his life. Starkweather's own mother told him to instead go to the electric chair, because it would shame the family to have someone labeled mentally unfit.

However, increasingly the public actually admires people when they courageously step forward and admit to human imperfection. First Lady Betty Ford became all the more admired when she publicly discussed her issues with alcohol and substance abuse. Many celebrities will attest to the outpouring of public support when they have gone public with their mental issues.

It simply is an outdated concept that being bipolar will make a family look "bad." Especially families who are familiar with generating publicity can find ways of presenting this information in a positive light.

Getting Your Priorities in Order

Having a sense of purpose in life involves behavior, as well as attitude. It is important to have a deep sense of purpose in life, but it will not come to much if you do not actually live with a sense of purpose.

This means having a clear idea of what your priorities are—what really matters and what does not.

If your moods are not stable, it is doubtful that anything else is going to be right. It may not be obvious today, but tomorrow or in two weeks, even things that seem to be going right might start to go wrong. You owe it to yourself, and to the people you are around, to make sure your mental state of being is as healthy as possible.

If your treatment is working, stick with it. Hopefully, you are one of the 60 percent of patients who find treatment that virtually eliminates future episodes, or at least dramatically minimizes them. If so, then keep up the good work. Even if everything else goes wrong that day, if you took your medication you got the most important thing right.

If you are still looking for the right treatment, keep looking. Unless your doctor thinks that the possibilities have been exhausted, you should keep trying different combinations. If you hear of a new medication, you should ask your doctor about it.

If you cannot take medication, do everything else you can. Get as much information from your doctor or other reliable sources as to how you can try to maintain stable moods as best as possible. Keep your eyes and ears open to alternative treatments, be in therapy or a support group—and also keep in mind the possibility of newer medications that might work for you.

(Self-)Honesty Is the Best Policy

So how are you really doing? How do you know if you are doing a better job of running your life? How do you know if you are genuinely connecting to other people? There are a number of steps you can take to find answers to these and other matters. But the main thing to remember is to be honest.

Develop a Checklist

Figure out what sorts of things you want to accomplish in a given day—or week, month, or year. These can be tangible goals, such as going back to school. But there can also be items on the checklist such as: "Am I eating (or sleeping) regularly?" Or: "Am I finishing one task before starting another one?" Or, for that matter: "When was the last time I felt suicidal?"

Each person is different, so each person might need a different checklist. This is something you might work on with your doctor. Figure out how mania and depression each tend to steer your life off course, and what sorts of things you can do each day to stay on track.

If you are basically doing these things each day—whether they are specific actions, or changes of attitude—you are probably on the right track. But the world's greatest checklist means nothing if you are not answering the questions honestly. If you ignore the reality of your life, no one will be fooled—including yourself. At the same time, you do not need to be your harshest critic. Do not put yourself down, or find fault just for the sake of finding fault. Instead, think in terms of "needs improvement" or "needs more work." But again, be honest.

Therapy

Everyone feels differently sometimes. It is normal to change your mind, to go from happy to sad, or to reinterpret a situation. It is even normal, yes, to be confused sometimes about who you are or what you want. But bipolar people experience such extreme fluctuations that the task of gaining self-knowledge can be all the more daunting.

If you are seeing a therapist, this should be helping you to get more in touch with the real you—what your happiness is and is not, your strengths and weaknesses, and how you perceive yourself through a day of life.

If you are feeling *more* uncertain and confused, you should tell your therapist about this. Perhaps this is a good thing, a phase in your personal development as you let go of some of your old assumptions. But it also might be that the therapy simply is not working, and that this is not the right therapist for you.

Sometimes, patients think they have developed crushes on their therapists. This is often called *transference*—the patient has projected his self-love onto the healer. In some respects, it can signal that the patient truly does want to get better, and is considered a normal part of the therapeutic process to work through. But in the case of bipolar people, these feelings can get out of control. If other kinds of feelings do start to develop, you should tell the therapist about it and ask if you should discontinue seeing him or her.

 ## Fact

Social learning theory posits that we learn how to behave by imitating others. For example, children will learn to be abusive or kind by watching how the adults around them behave. This process of basing your behavior on what you have seen others do is called modeling.

Honesty with Others

In general, people in this society have trouble with honesty. Some think that it is rude to ever share anything sad or unpleasant, while others have the opposite problem, and think everything they say must be negative or else it is not the truth. Knowing how to say things that are accurate, and in just the right way, is a learned skill—a balancing act that will sometimes fail, no matter who you are.

Possibly the question people ask of each other most often is: "How are you?" And probably the most common response is: "Fine." It is polite small talk; often the asker does not really care how the other person is. Just as often, the responder is not really fine, but figures that "fine" is the expected answer.

However, for a bipolar individual, "How are you?" can be an important question. There is nothing harmful in polite small talk. But somewhere along the way, there should be people in your life with whom you can share that you are *not* fine, if such is the case. In fact, if you feel yourself veering close to depression, it can be extremely useful to connect to someone. And of course, you should tell your psychiatrist.

On the other hand, if you are teetering on a manic episode, you might be unable to *stop* talking. Once again, it is of utmost importance that your psychiatrist be aware of your mood. And other people in your life can be told to recognize the warning signs, and encourage you to get additional help.

Alert

Many people do not realize that self-disclosure is a selective process. No one ever tells another person "everything" about herself. Even the closest of relationships involve at least some secrecy. Just because someone tells you one of her secrets, it does not mean she has told you everything there is to know.

But short of mania, find someone whose communication style you admire, and study what she does. You will probably find that this person does not take longer than necessary to make a certain point, and lets others into the conversation. She can express being angry, for example, without creating the impression that something violent is about to happen.

The middle road might feel unfamiliar, but after a while it can feel like home.

Learning to Problem-Solve

It is extremely useful to approach problems logically, and with a certain amount of detachment. In this way, problems do not have to be overwhelming. They can even seem like interesting challenges.

Break Down the Problem

Let's say you either do not drive or else do not have a car. There is no bus service in your community. You need to get to the drugstore way across town to pick up a prescription. A friend agreed to get it for you, but then your friend leaves a message saying that he cannot run the errand, after all. There is no one else who lives in town that you feel comfortable calling.

You can get upset because the problem seems "impossible" to solve, and you are scared of what might happen if you do not get your medication in time. Or, you can break down the problem into a series of steps:

1. Are you *sure* there is no one else you can call to run the errand as a favor?
2. Can you offer to pay someone a few dollars for his time—or if you are broke, to give him an IOU to dinner or a movie?
3. If still no one is available, is there a local cab company? (Probably there is.) If you think it will be "too expensive," is there something else you can do without?
4. If there is no cab, how far is it to walk? Would walking for, say, an hour or so this one time really be *that* bad?
5. To avoid this situation in the future, are you sure there are no social services or charities available that could provide transportation or run the errand for you once a month? Check with your public library, police department, city hall, or place of worship to try to find out.

Rather than letting yourself feel hopeless and upset, it is possible to logically think about what to do, step by step. The problem need not seem to be more than you can handle.

Produce More Than One Solution

Critical thinking is the ability to look at a situation from more than one point of view. Answers to problems do not fall from the sky; they are created and enacted through human endeavor. Thus, it is usually a mistake to think in terms of finding *the* one possible, great, eternal answer. Both for your peace of mind and for practical considerations, it is a good idea to always have a Plan B—or even Plan C.

For instance, using the same example of needing a ride to the drugstore: If you call for a cab, make sure you leave enough time to get there some other way—even if it means walking for an hour. If it turns out there is a special shuttle service for people with disabilities, by all means arrange to use it. But maybe you can also call your friend back and say, "I have made arrangements so that I will not have to take advantage of your generosity anymore. But just in case the shuttle can't make it one day, is it still okay if I ask for your help?"

Rather than frantically trying to convince yourself that you should not be worried about things going wrong, take that nervous energy and put it to good use by developing a Plan B. This should lessen your anxiety.

Remember the Big Picture

From time to time, everyone makes a proverbial mountain out of a molehill. Something that does not matter very much is treated as though the fate of the world depended on it. However, for bipolar people, losing a sense of perspective can inspire dramatic shifts of mood.

It is a good idea to keep the problems of everyday life in perspective. Again, using the same example: Was it *that* big a deal that you were inconvenienced for maybe an extra hour or so in order to get your medication? If you got angry at your friend for letting you down, what if he really couldn't help it? What if you were living in a time or place in which your medication was not even available? What if you were one of those less fortunate people who do not respond to medication?

 Fact

Attribution theory explores how people attribute certain results to certain circumstances. Generally, people believe they earn their successes, and that their failures result from outside circumstances—that it was not their fault that they failed. When it comes to others, people often think that they do not deserve their successes, but that they do deserve their failures. This is called the fundamental attribution error.

Additionally, you might consider: Are there other things you did during your day that *did* go according to plan? Did you feel good about something else you did? What are your long-range goals, and in general are you making progress toward achieving them?

In these and other ways, you can not only deal with a given problem at hand, but also keep it in perspective by remembering the big picture of your life.

Spirituality, or Something Similar

There are people who claim to be not at all spiritual and to also have happy and rewarding lives. It is not necessary to be spiritual if you want to maximize your chances for mental harmony. But whether it is spirituality or something else, it can be extremely useful to have some kind of belief system—some sense of what you are living for. Perhaps you already have something that works for you. But for those who do not, here are some ways to start looking.

Religious Versus Spiritual

To be *religious* is to belong to an organized body that worships on a regular basis. If you want constancy in your life, and want to connect to a regular group of people, you might find that an organized religion is a good thing to try. On the other hand, some people find any one religion too confining. They want more variety, and more exposure to different schools of thought. So they may join more than one religion.

But another possibility is to consider yourself *spiritual*. This means you do not really join any one religion, but look for spiritual meaning from every possible source. This has the advantage of offering the possibility of exposure to a wide range of people and teachings. On the other hand, some people do not find there is enough structure or foundation in simply being spiritual. Again, the choice is yours.

But whether you choose to be religious or spiritual, you have the opportunity to be exposed to a body of teachings that offers an explanation for the reason for existence, a set of guideposts to live by, and reminders that the things that matter most in life often lie beyond the surface. Both spirituality and religion also give you the chance to meet other people who are trying to live on a deeper level.

L. Essential

About 60 percent of Americans specifically believe in God, and over 90 percent more generally in God or some other form of universal spirit. At the same time, over 50 percent of all Americans believe that God rewards good earthly deeds, regardless of religion. And about 45 percent of Americans believe an atheist can "go to heaven" if he or she lives a good life.

However, if neither religion nor spirituality works for you, there are many non-religious, or secular belief systems as well.

Secular Humanism

One of the most popular non-religious philosophies is secular humanism. (It is possible to be both religious [or spiritual] *and* a secular humanist, but some people are only the latter.) The basic premise of secular humanism is that the greatest thing anyone can do is to help other people—that life does not get any more "spiritual" than this, and that there is no higher purpose than this. Energy that could otherwise go into worship for the sake of worship is instead spent on social activism, such as:

- Helping people with physical, mental or economic disadvantages
- Working for fair laws and social justice for all people
- Protecting the environment
- Improving your local community

The sense of reward and purpose you may feel from such activities is believed to be its own reward. Many people find that their own problems become less important when they practice secular humanism.

Though some religions are concerned that too much secular humanism will dilute their spiritual purpose, many embrace it as part of the purpose of their religion. And in any case, virtually all religions engage in some acts of charity.

Finding Meaning in Being Bipolar

Most anyone can benefit from religion, spirituality, and/or secular humanism. However, bipolar people might specifically gain from seeing their disorder in terms of a larger purpose in life:

- If your treatment is working, can you share your story with others and encourage them to get the help they need?
- Can the hardships you have experienced as a bipolar person be used to give you more empathy for the struggles of other people, whatever their problems?
- Do you feel you understand more about the human condition for having endured bipolar episodes?
- Since you are not just a bipolar person but many other things as well, can you devote some amount of time or energy to making the world a better place—whatever that means to you?

These are just some of the questions you can ask yourself in trying to bring more meaning and purpose into your life.

Managing Mania

Even if you have been responding well to mood stabilizers, it is possible that you will find yourself edging toward hypomania—or even full-scale mania. Perhaps something specific has happened that is making you become highly agitated. Or maybe your mood stabilizers are not 100 percent effective. In any case, are there things you can do to try to slow yourself down and maintain a more balanced pace? This chapter answers this and many other questions you may still have.

Be Prepared

No matter how long it has been since you had a hypomanic or manic episode, there is always a possibility that you will have one again. At the same time, just because you are a bit on edge or had to stay up late to finish a project, it does not necessarily mean you are verging on mania. Still, it is important to be aware that certain kinds of situations might increase the likelihood of mania. Besides knowing specifics about your own situation, there are some general ideas to keep in mind.

Stay Out of the Fast Lane

From time to time, everyone is rushed—especially in today's fast-paced world. There will be days in which you cannot avoid having to do several things at once, as quickly as possible. You might have to hurry to a store before it closes—only your car desperately needs gas. Or your boss is counting on you to finish a report by noon, and you have other work that needs to get done the same day. Or you are cooking Thanksgiving dinner for your entire family, which can stress out *anybody*. However, you can still try to live your life as sensibly as possible:

- **Try to avoid highly stressful jobs.** For example, if a job involves a lot of last-minute deadlines, or waiting on large numbers of people who all want service immediately, it might not be the job for you. Even if the job seems relatively low key, if it turns out there is a boss or employee who makes everyone extremely angry, it might likewise not be a good environment for a bipolar person.
- **By contrast, a job in which you have relative freedom to pace yourself,** is flexible and offers frequent short breaks, and either is staffed by kind people or else gives you relative autonomy, might be much better for you.
- **Try to avoid situations that are likely to be high stress.** You do not have to offer to perform certain tasks, errands, or favors that either someone else can do, or else do not really need to get done.
- **Ask for help when appropriate.** If you do volunteer to cook Thanksgiving dinner, or take on some difficult task at work, ask for help. The only reason not to would be if, for example, the job situation is one in which you literally cannot ask for help. But if something can be a team effort, it will probably stress you out less.
- **Pace yourself.** Take short breaks whenever possible. Step outside and get some fresh air. Have a snack. Read a few more pages of a book, listen to some music, or take some deep breaths. Keep an active awareness of the world around you, and remember that the task you are performing is only so important.
- **Avoid putting things off until the last minute.** If you can do a little bit of a job on one day, a little bit more the next, you can avoid having to rush around at the last minute to meet a deadline. This can keep you from feeling as stressed.

Fact

Stress costs the U.S. workplace some $300 billion each year. This figure includes compensation claims related to stress, health insurance and medical costs, absenteeism, employee turnover, and reduced productivity. Upward of 40 percent of the workers who experience job burnout claim that stress is the main problem.

Pay Attention to the Calendar

Certain dates might be more associated with a manic episode than others. These can include the following:

- **Cycles:** If your history of manic (or depressive) episodes tends to run in cycles, maintain an active awareness of these patterns. For example, if your mania used to follow your depression, and you just got done feeling slightly depressed, you should be prepared for the possibility that you now might likewise feel at least slightly manic.
- **Seasons:** As previously mentioned in Chapter 5, seasonal changes are sometimes associated with dramatic mood swings in bipolar people. The warmer seasons tend to be associated with mania, and the cooler seasons tend to be associated with depression.
- **Anniversaries:** The anniversary of a major life event potentially can trigger a manic episode. This is especially likely when the event is associated with a loss of some kind, such as divorce, the death of a loved one, or other kinds of disruptions. Also, anniversaries of major episodes can be a vulnerable time. In all of these instances, unprocessed memories of the emotions felt at the time can bring forth an episode.
- **Forthcoming events:** Whether it is something stressful (such as a court date) or something potentially highly positive

(such as a marriage or promotion at work), any sort of major change can set in motion a manic episode. So it is good to discuss in advance with your doctor how to deal with this forthcoming event.

Alert

Among non-bipolar people, anniversaries of sad or traumatic occasions are much more likely to be associated with depression. If an undiagnosed person responds to, say, the anniversary of the death of a beloved spouse with energy frenetic enough to seem manic, it might be that this person should see a doctor.

Warning Signals

Whatever you are doing or not doing in your daily life, there are some general warning signals that you should heed. Otherwise, you might be teetering on a manic episode.

There are a number of areas in which you can monitor yourself for marked changed in a more manic direction:

- **Speech patterns:** Are you talking more rapidly than normal? Are you having trouble not talking? Is your voice louder than usual? Are you getting hoarse more often? If you are not face-to-face with others, do you feel compelled to write a letter, send an e-mail, or talk on the phone so that you can keep communicating nonstop?
- **Eating and sleeping:** Are your eating and/or sleeping patterns dramatically changing?
- **Busy without productivity:** Are you seemingly always active, yet accomplishing very little? Do some of the tasks you take on have no purpose?

- **Irritability:** Are you more easily irritated than usual? Do small things annoy you more than they usually do?
- **Feeling threatened:** If you do not get your own way or are interrupted, do you feel much more threatened and hostile than usual? Do you find yourself wanting to argue with people much more than you usually do?
- **Lavishness:** Are you suddenly spending more money, giving more gifts, and/or taking more trips? Are you suddenly living beyond your means?
- **Interference:** Are you suddenly giving people advice whether they want it or not? Do you feel like you are being exceptionally generous as you do so, as though you are a superior person bestowing wisdom upon a lesser being?
- **Behavior with strangers:** Are you suddenly overly friendly, generous, or nosy toward people you do not even know? Are you asking inappropriate questions of strangers, or engaging in high-risk behavior with them (including sex)?
- **Heightened drama:** In general, are you feeling more of a need to stand out from the crowd—to talk, act, or dress differently— in a way that makes everyone notice you? Whether angry or happy, is the feeling suddenly more intense—as though you'll never stop being angry, or never stop laughing?

Another general type of warning can come from other people, be they loved ones or other kinds of contacts. At the most basic and significant level, your doctor might tell you that you seem much more agitated or hyper, or that you are speaking more rapidly, or displaying other symptoms that make for serious concern.

People who care about you and are familiar with your diagnosis might also tell you that you seem to be edging toward an episode. They might put it in the form of a question, such as: "Do you think you are having serious problems?" or "Have you talked to your doctor about the way you are acting?" Or they might simply comment that you seem much more agitated, and should get some extra help. In any case, this feedback is probably worth taking seriously.

L. Essential

People you have just been introduced to might also give you valuable input. If you go too far with them, they might tell you to go away, stop asking them questions, stop trying to buy them drinks, etc. The encounter might quickly escalate to shouting, or even violence. At the other extreme, a stranger might tell you that you are the friendliest person they ever met, or the funniest or smartest. All these are clues you can evaluate in terms of your condition.

Furthermore, people whom you know, but who do not know you are bipolar, might notice that something seems wrong and say things like: "You seem on edge lately," or "Did something happen that I don't know about, because all of a sudden you have a very short fuse." They also might express naïve puzzlement over something you did, such as how you were able to afford something you bought, or since when do you pick up strangers in bars, or how they never knew you were such an angry or funny person. People you work with might wonder aloud why you did not finish your work as you normally do, or that you must have stayed up all night getting something done in record time.

Protect Your Personal Life

If you should veer off into the world of mania, there are a number of precautionary steps you can take to keep your personal life intact. Hopefully, you will get the help you need before things digress too far. But however far things go, here are some things you can do to try to minimize the negative consequences to you and your loved ones.

Preparing Your Loved Ones

Hopefully, your immediate loved ones—such as your spouse and children—are aware you're bipolar, and also aware of what that means. It is important that these people have been given your own account of the situation and how the disorder affects you personally; a list of warning signs so your loved ones will now what to watch for; a clear sense that they did not cause you to become afflicted with the disorder; and outside resources, including the contact information for your doctor(s), support groups, and other persons who have a bipolar loved one.

The Aftermath

Whether you simply went slightly off course or had a full-blown episode, once your moods are stabilized again you should not take your loved ones for granted. Group counseling might be appropriate, at least for the short term. In any event, talk to your doctor as to the most appropriate way of handling each loved one.

If you consciously chose to go off your medication, some sort of explanation and/or apology might well be in order. Should the episode have happened despite all your best intentions, you still will want to not only share how it was for you, but also let your loved ones share what it was like for them.

Do not assume you know how your loved ones feel, or what it was like for them. Ask them, and let them tell you in their own words. Even if you are tempted, avoid responding defensively, correcting their experiences, or keeping the focus solely on yourself. Again, this is where a professional can moderate the discussion, and keep it on track.

What If You Have Done Things You Regret?

Hopefully, you did not do anything so dramatic that it cannot be undone. This is not to trivialize that your loved ones might have had their feelings hurt, been embarrassed or humiliated, or been frightened for themselves or for you. But if you did not have an affair, leave your spouse, deplete the family savings, quit your job, sell the house, disown a child . . . if your mania did not advance to these kinds of heightened states, you hopefully will be able to get past whatever happened with time and effort.

However, if you did do something truly drastic, you need to realize that the person or people you hurt may not be able to let you back in their lives—or at least not for a while. Often, dramatic changes work against mood stabilization. But if, for example, your spouse has decided to leave you—or you left him or her while you were manic—you might need to accept this change as best as you can, with your doctor's help.

If your inner circle is essentially still intact, despite what you did— if, for example, your spouse wants you back—you need to seriously think about what you can do to try to ensure that you do not have another major episode. Talk to your doctor about it. If it appears that there is little you can do to prevent future episodes, you and your spouse need to communicate deeply about how to proceed—preferably in the presence of a doctor or therapist.

Protect Your Assets

There are numerous steps you can take to try to minimize any damage to your finances, property, or other assets, should you have a manic episode. Ironically, the more you have, the more you can do to protect yourself—therefore, the less you have, the more you can lose. But whether rich or poor, you might find the following steps useful.

Pay for Safety

If you are at least moderately well off, you might find it worthwhile to make a few expenditures as insurance against losing virtually everything. For instance, talk to professionals. Consult with an attorney about matters such as requiring the co-signature of a spouse—or even a disinterested third party—before you can spend, sell, trade, or give away past a certain amount. Such consultations might also involve an accountant, banker, or stockbroker.

You can also set up an allowance. With an attorney and accountant, you can agree to have access to only so much money per week. This could also be so much per month or year, but probably smaller amounts accessed over shorter time periods will lessen the possibility of large-scale irresponsible spending.

Finally, create an advance directive. This involves a signed legal document in which the bipolar person gives permission for another individual (such as a doctor or family member) to ensure you receive proper treatment—even hospitalization—should you have another episode.

Limit Your Liquid Assets

If most of your finances are tied up in investments that you cannot access without third-party intervention, there are fewer liquid assets for you to waste in a frenzy of mania. If you have credit cards at all, they should have relatively low credit limits—as well as reasonable interest rates.

If you have a checking account, make it a joint account with a trusted third party who has power of attorney. That way, if you seem to be out of control, this other person can close out the account. (You can also set up the account to require joint signatures on all checks, though this can be extremely inconvenient.) At many banks, you can set up your checking account to have protections in place to cover overdrafts. But you should also set limits on this process, such as making most of your savings unavailable to cover overdrafts at any given time.

Talk to your banker about other steps you can take to limit your liquid assets. He or she will be a professional whom you should be able to trust. But you probably will not need to share very much about why you want certain precautionary measures in place; the main point will be that you *do.*

What If You Do Not Have Much to Start With?

Millions of people in the United States now live one paycheck away from homelessness—they have no savings, no property, and no valuable heirlooms. If you are one of these people, it is difficult to afford lengthy consultations with attorneys.

But you can see if there are inexpensive or even free legal services in your community. If you are a college student, there might be a legal aid service provided, particularly if there is a law school. There are also law libraries that provide examples of different kinds of legal documents. You can also consult online links for such examples, including *http://ppc.uslegalforms.com* and *www.legalzoom.com*. While an attorney should still look these over, you can do at least some of the work yourself.

Also, you can still avoid having access to a great many credit cards, or a limit that is higher than you can afford. And you can still have some safety precautions in place on any bank account that you do have.

 Alert

In today's world, bipolar people are hardly the only ones who spend beyond their means. At present, the credit-card debt in the United States is in the neighborhood of $560 billion. The average American household can claim a credit card debt of about $11,000.

If you bounce checks in a fit of mania, you will be faced with high overdraft charges. You might need to face the reality that any check you write should have a co-signature. Or maybe you should not have checks or credit cards, and should only deal with whatever cash you have on hand. (In this case, you should still always get a bank check or money order when paying rent or other important bills, so that there is documented proof.)

Protect Your Professional Life

If you have a job, you do not want to jeopardize it, or cause problems for your coworkers or clients while in the throes of mania. Here are some steps you can take to try to protect yourself professionally.

Allow for Missing Work

If you are becoming manic, it might be in your best interests to take a few sick or vacation days until your mood can be stabilized. Ideally, your employer is aware of your condition and will understand. However, some people put themselves in positions whereby if they miss work, the rest of the enterprise can barely function. It is nice to be considered important, but if you are bipolar you might want to avoid the pressure of being quite so indispensable. Hopefully, there is at least one other person who can do what you do.

Still other people are in work environments in which the general environment makes it hard to take time off. People who miss work at all get fired, or at the very least become the boss's enemy. Again, try to avoid working at such a place. You need to have some flexibility in case you experience an episode.

If you are self-employed, try not to be in a position in which you cannot survive without a sale or a check from a client within a given week. Hopefully, you have enough assets to fall back on so that you can take a day or two off here and there to attend to your mental health. If you are in business with someone else, ask that person to fill in for you, and make it up to him or her with money or in some other way.

If Work Cannot Be Avoided

If people are depending on you to finish or do something by a certain date—or if to *not* do it for any reason would be to commit professional suicide—you should talk to your doctor about what steps you can take to minimize the onslaught of mania. Even here, your mental health should ultimately come first. But there are some things you can do in the meantime:

- **Pace yourself as best you can.** Whatever it is, hopefully you can still take breaks, get at least a few minutes of fresh air, and remember to eat and sleep.
- **Take steps to counter the high energy.** When you are done working at the end of the day, take a long hot bath, meditate,

read or watch TV in bed, or do whatever you need to do to calm down.

- **Stay in close communication with your doctor.** Let him or her know of any increase in your manic symptoms.
- **Communicate with loved ones.** Let those closest to you know what is going on, and what they might be able to do to help.

Become Your Own Parent

Just like a good parent takes care of her child through good times and bad, the wise bipolar person learns to attend to her illness, celebrating the good times, weathering the bad, but never giving up. Above all, you must always take responsibility for your situation. Though you can benefit immensely from support and feedback from others, in the final analysis, you and only you experience your moods first-hand. Whether you realize it or not, you know quite a lot about what sorts of situations challenge your mood stability.

 Question

Should bipolar adults avoid going back to school since it would represent a big life change?
Absolutely not! About 50 percent of the people who attend graduate school are older, non-traditional students who have been out of school for some time. Characteristically, such students report that education means more to them than it did when they were younger, and they do quite well.

You may need to parent yourself sometimes, and say to yourself (or to other people) that unfortunately, you cannot go to that party, have that extramarital affair, go to that family reunion, or work late at the office—if you know that there is a good chance doing this thing will set in motion mood swings. You may have to disappoint yourself—or other people—but your mental equilibrium needs to come first. If anniversaries, seasonal changes, or other events or times tend to be difficult for you, remember to plan ahead. Keep your doctor appointments, and take your medication, no matter what else is going right or wrong. A good parent keeps feeding and sheltering its young, regardless of what else is going on. At the same basic level, you should stay on your treatment program—period.

Furthermore, just as a parent might never give up on his child, a bipolar person can have the attitude of never giving up. Even if there are some unexpected crises along the way, even if medication does not seem to help, and even if sometimes it all just seems like too much to bother with anymore, you can keep at it. Tomorrow might bring a new kind of treatment that works better. Or your present crisis might start to go away.

Even if in the past you have not been able to hold down a job, some new kind of work opportunity might come along that you can handle. Maybe it means going back to school. If in the past you could not sustain intimate relationships—or even friendships—maybe starting today you *will* be able to. The point is to remember that some days are bound to feel better than others. But part of taking responsibility for your situation is never giving up on yourself.

CHAPTER 13

Dealing with Depression

Just as you might unexpectedly find yourself speeding toward mania, you might also start slowing down into depression. It is just as important to find constructive ways of keeping depression at bay as it is to resist mania. At the same time, since everyone feels unhappy sometimes, it is important to distinguish between a normal range of sorrow and serious, chronic depression. This chapter includes some steps you can take.

Sadness, Mild Depression, and Chronic Depression

Everyone is unhappy sometimes. Sometimes upsetting events are shown in the news or you hear about them from a friend. Or maybe an individual is reminded of something from the past—or feels uncertain about the future. There are even times in which the average person feels unhappy without knowing why. But there is a difference between sadness and depression—just as there is a difference between mild and severe depression.

Sadness

It is perfectly normal to feel sad over a wide range of small or large events. The virtually endless list of things that often make people sad would include: when a relationship ends, a job ends, a school year ends, you lose money, you lose a minor court case, your favorite team loses the Super Bowl, your favorite movie star loses the Oscar, your pet dies, your country is at war, the news announces that a child was murdered, waxing nostalgic over the past . . . sadness is likely to touch most people's lives on a fairly regular basis.

This type of sadness is a normal response that does not keep people from functioning in other ways. In fact, it often is cleansing to have what is called a "good cry," or to listen to a favorite sad song. If people were never sad, being happy would not mean very much. Sadness can humble people, and reminds them of what is really important in their lives. It has often been said that without a healthy dose of sadness now and then, people cannot mature, or have compassion for others.

 Alert

Sadness is not depression. Sadness does not cause you to lose interest in people and activities, nor does it make you unable to leave the house, or make even the smallest of decisions with confidence. It does not wreak havoc upon your eating and sleeping patterns. Most important of all, sadness does not make you suicidal and obsessed with death.

There is a world of difference between sadness and depression. If a bipolar person feels sad now and then, she is just being a normal person. In fact, it might even signal a healthy mental outlook, since it is absolutely appropriate to feel sad over certain things that happen. If you are bipolar and are feeling what has sometimes been called "blue," you need to determine if you simply are sad, or if you are experiencing depression. And by all means discuss your moods with your doctor, to make sure.

Mild and Chronic Depression

The basic symptoms of depression have already been outlined. More minor forms of depression often happen over specific incidents.

The depression might also be a painful reminder of something from the person's past. While quite painful for the person who is depressed, such depression often passes when the situation is resolved. Therapy is helpful for getting at the root cause of the unhappiness; antidepressants might be prescribed on a short- or long-term basis.

People suffering from mild depression can still function, but they do so half-heartedly. They merely are going through the motions, and their minds seem to be somewhere else, even when they technically smile or laugh. Still, they are able to get by until the feeling passes.

Chronic depression can still benefit from therapy, but quite often there is a physiological basis for it. It comes and goes without anything to necessarily trigger it. For bipolar people—as well as unipolar people—this is where long-term usage of antidepressants comes into play. Chronic depression goes way beyond sadness. For example, let's say someone has just broken off a serious relationship. If merely sad, the person might strangely enjoy listening to his ex's favorite song, because it brings up sentimental—if sorrowful—feelings that are a kind of balm to the soul. However, if depressed, this person would not be able to stand hearing this song. The painful heaviness inside seems to intensify unbearably at the mere thought of it. In fact, it might be so painful that death might seem the only way to escape from it. You do not have a "good cry," but instead might cry uncontrollably, without anything specific causing it.

Essential

For many people, depression comes and goes, but on any day of the week there will always be many people who are depressed. In fact, at least 5 percent of the total U.S. population is always seriously depressed at any given point in time.

Depression, especially chronic depression, is *not* about feeling a little sorry for yourself, or being a "drama queen." It is not something you can just snap out of by remembering an upbeat saying, or forcing yourself to smile.

Preventing Depression

Serious depression can be extremely difficult to control, and it is important to stay in close contact with your doctor and/or therapist if you are chronically depressed. Still, as with mania, you can try to minimize the likelihood of a depressive episode by taking certain practical measures in your daily life.

Healthy Mind and Body

Fresh air, exercise, and a balanced diet can help you to feel good about yourself. Besides the benefits of having a well body, these are ways of telling yourself that you deserve to be treated well—you deserve fresh air, sunshine, good food, and a refreshed body. But try to make it all fun. For example, rather than force yourself to go outside, what is something you enjoy doing outdoors? If you truly hate going to a gym, is there some other form of exercise—even just taking long walks—that gives you pleasure? Maybe you do not like Brussels sprouts or cauliflower, but are there fruits and vegetables you do enjoy?

Many people benefit from taking up yoga or meditation, or other relaxation techniques. If you cannot afford classes, you can probably find books or tapes in your public library on these topics.

A Well-Paced Life

Try not to do either too much or too little. If you are pushing yourself too hard, you might become unhappy—especially if things go wrong after all your effort. You also might wear down your immune system, and make yourself vulnerable to physical illness.

But at the same time, doing utterly nothing day after day can make *anyone* depressed. If you are unable to work outside the home, perhaps there is work you could do within the home. Or if unable to work at all, you might still be able to take up a craft or hobby that engages your attention. If money is an issue, then if nothing else there is the public library—become well read, or an expert on a given topic. Set a goal such as reading the complete works of a certain author.

Still another area to consider is volunteer work. You might meet some nice people while doing something that helps society—and reminds you of a deeper purpose for living.

A steady, non-chaotic daily life can bring steadiness and clarity. But at the same time, you do not want to feel bored. If you work, plan interesting evenings, weekends, and vacations. If your finances are limited, even just driving or walking to town—or taking the bus—can add interest to your life. There might be unfamiliar neighborhoods in your town you can explore, as well.

 Fact

Even though a solid 80 percent of the people who seek treatment for depression find improvement, two-thirds of the people who are afflicted by depression do not seek treatment. Their depression not only keeps them from accomplishing all they could, but affects the people they know and love.

If you watch TV, select whatever shows you most want to watch, even if other people might think you made a silly choice. It is your time, your TV, your life. Nonetheless, you might avoid watching anything that might be too disturbing for you to handle. For example, if there is a news program about some real-life tragedy that sounds depressing, you might not be up to watching it.

A Happy Home

You will want your home environment—and your work environment, if applicable—to be as unlikely as possible to contribute to a depressed stated of mind. There are number of simple things you can do to help.

Keep It Cheerful and Clean

As previously discussed, a tranquil home can help you to feel stable and good about yourself. Clutter and filth tend to make people unhappy. If possible, have at least one object in each room of your home that makes you happy when you see it. If nothing else, just being in a place of order and clean smells can make even a threadbare room seem more attractive and pleasant.

Bright, warm colors (such as yellow, orange, and red) tend to make people happy, so you might want to paint your walls something cheerful. If that is not possible, you can see about hanging happy-looking pictures or tapestries on the walls.

Some people find that simple touches, such as candles, incense, plants, flowers, or a bowl of fresh fruit, also help make a room feel happy. If something is broken, either get it fixed or throw it away; reminders of broken objects are depressing for some people. If certain music makes you unhappy, do not keep it in your house. The same holds true for books, pictures, or DVDs.

Your bed and bedding should be comfortable. Some people never quite get around to replacing their lumpy mattress, scratchy blankets, or limp old pillows—and then wonder why they never feel truly rested after sleeping. Even if you do not have a lot of money, a comfortable bed is a wise investment—even if you have to buy a refurbished mattress second-hand.

Keep reminders of happy times around your home: photos of people you care about, of happy occasions; or other objects that stir pleasant memories and remind you of *not* being depressed.

Clear Away Bad Memories

You should not be reminded of painful memories on a regular basis. For example, if you feel unhappy whenever you think of a certain person, do not keep her portrait on display in your home (or office). If old scrapbooks or other kinds of souvenirs likewise have a deeply upsetting effect, keep them boxed away, even in a storage facility, if you can afford it. Should you tend to be a "pack rat," you might want to consider changing your ways. If *all* some old memento does is make you unhappy, it is not against the law to part with it.

L. Essential

Depression has been estimated to cost the United States over $30 billion a year. This figure includes factors such as lost work and income, and medical, legal, and criminal situations that emerge around untreated depression. It is in the best interest of society at large to educate people on the symptoms of depression, and the many resources available to deal with it.

If your parents make you unhappy and they have given you their old furniture, it might just be worth your while to part with it. If you can afford new furniture (even used furniture), there probably is no reason why you should not have it. Should money be an issue, you can at least refurbish the pieces to give them your own look—something that says *you* instead of them. You might also consider simply doing without a lot of things, if that's what it takes to feel good about yourself.

If there is someone from the past whom you do not like hearing from, screen your phone calls. If possible, you can get a new, unlisted number and not give it to this person.

What to Do If You're Depressed

If you do start to feel unhappy, and you recognize it to be depression and not merely sadness, there are number of things you can do to try to steer yourself away from it. Take a proactive stance before the depression becomes overwhelming, and use all the tools at your disposal to fight against it. These can include the obvious, such as your doctor. But there are other methods of empowerment that you can employ, including:

- **Learn the signs.** If certain thoughts or moods have signaled the onslaught of depression in the past, recognize them for what they are in the present.
- **Know what works.** If talking to certain people, watching a certain video, or reading a certain book has worked before to keep you from getting depressed, by all means do the same thing again.
- **Find people who cheer you up.** If you know people who are good listeners and who have a great deal of empathy to offer when you are feeling out of sorts, by all means talk to them. If other people usually do not cheer you up, talk to them only as a last resort. For example, maybe you think a mother is "supposed to" make her children feel better, but if in reality yours often makes you feel worse, stick to more upbeat people. You can always talk to your mother again when you are feeling better.
- **Build a formal support system.** Maybe you are part of a local support group, or have an online support group. By all means use these contacts when you feel yourself veering toward depression.

Continuing to behave in regular, healthy ways can also help with depression. For example, keep regular sleeping habits. If you are physically exhausted, by all means take a nap; it might be just what you need. But if you are sleeping for days on end to escape from the world, this will only reinforce the oncoming depression. It also can render you unable to sleep at night, which likewise can foster depression.

Also keep up your daily responsibilities. Though it might be tempting to take an early vacation—or even quit your job—try to resist. Feeling connected to the outside world will help. Even if you do not work, give yourself errands to run, and people to go see.

Another wise thing to do is avoid negativity whenever possible. Avoid people, places, and things that tend to bring you down. If in your own mind you are seeing everything as negative, talk to your doctor about how you can learn to remember to see the good side of things as well.

 ## Question

Can writing help alleviate feelings of depression?
Yes. Whether it is simply to vent or to create something of interest to other people, use your unhappy thoughts creatively by writing them down. This can be a journal, or it can be a poem, story, play, or novel. The sheer act of writing will distract your mind away from the depression, and the insights you discover may make you feel happy.

Finally, go outside and get some fresh air. Even if you have to force yourself, even if it is cold or wet, experience the elements for even just a few minutes. Look up at the sky; take in the sights and sounds and smells. If it is a nice day, sit outside and read, if nothing else.

If Depression Escalates

If despite whatever you did or did not do, you find your depression escalating, there are a number of things you can still do to protect yourself from doing anything you will regret. Reach out to providers of support, such as the following:

- **Your friends or loved ones:** If you are having a serious episode of depression, in addition to your doctor, people who care about you might be able to help out. If you live alone, it might be a good idea to see if you can sleep at a friend's house for the night. The sheer novelty might be refreshing, and maybe your friend can cheer you up. If you are a single parent, perhaps a relative or friend can help temporarily with your children.

- **Your doctor:** Most psychiatrists have an emergency number, or a switchboard that will forward emergency information. While waiting to talk to your doctor, you could also try your psychologist, or the facilitator of your weekly support group. If you cannot reach your psychiatrist, you can try your regular medical doctor. Ideally, you will have worked out ahead of time an arrangement with your psychiatrist should he go out of town.

- **Suicide hotline:** Most communities have a number you can call to speak to someone over the phone if you feel you might kill yourself. You can also call 1-800-SUICIDE (1-800-784-2433), or go online at: *http://suicidehotlines.com/national.html*.

- **911:** If need be, you can call 911 or another general emergency number, and explain that you are feeling dangerously depressed.

- **A hospital:** Another possibility is to check in to a hospital. Many medical hospitals have psychiatric wards; those that do not might still be able to send you over to one that does.

Depression is ruthless. It takes away your reason for living—and in so doing makes you not even want to bother to ask for help. You start to feel hopeless, as if nothing could possibly make this feeling go away. And if the hopelessness doesn't get to you, the accompanying feelings of unworthiness might. So that even if you did think help was possible, you might also think that no one wants to help you, no one cares, and if you *do* ask for help, all anyone will be is inconvenienced. Even worse, you might wrongly decide that no one will miss you when you're gone—or that even if a *few* people would, they somehow are not people who really matter.

Sadly, each year thousands of people reach this point where they do not ask for help—and many of them succeed in taking their lives. Do not become the next statistic. If it helps, consider the tables turned: What if someone came to *you* and said, "Help me, I think I might kill myself." Is there anyone, even your worst enemy, whom you would not try to help? Anyone whom you would not think it a waste to find out that they took their own life because of depression? You *are* worth saving. You *do* deserve to find the help you need.

⌷. Essential

It is estimated that more people suffer from depression than ever before. The average person is ten times more likely to experience depression now than fifty years ago. Possible explanations for this include more pressure on the average person to achieve lofty goals, and people taking less time to cultivate strong social bonds with others.

If you are calling up loved ones in the middle of the night on a regular basis, you probably need more help than they can give you. But if just every now and then you need someone to cheer you up or keep you company, you need not feel guilty for asking. *Even if people turn you down, it does not mean you should never have asked them.*

As for professionals: By definition, it is the *job* of mental professionals to help people who need it. So you should never feel guilty about turning to professional services when you need them. Depression can make people want to be isolated, but if you can just hit one button on your phone and speed dial a helpful source (having already input these numbers), you can get some serious help with minimal effort.

The Light at the End of the Tunnel

In the throes of depression, it is all too easy to feel that the heavy weight inside you will never lift. Difficult as it can be, try to remember other kinds of ideas. For example, focus on the other times in your life in which depression—or other problems—seemed insurmountable. Whatever it was, it seemed like you would never be able to stop obsessing about it, and the gloom would never lift for a moment.

Yet, through medication, therapy, your support network, and/or a simple twist of fate, whatever it was *did* go away. You no longer feel that same pain. You can recall that you felt bad, but it seems far away, and a little hard to relate to.

 ## Fact

Depression is the leading mental disorder in the world. Some sources have predicted that within the early twenty-first century, it will be second only to heart disease as a disabler of humankind. Globally, for all the new knowledge and technology to help people live easier or better lives, people are finding it more difficult to be happy.

As a bipolar person, you perhaps understand better than other people a simple fact of life: Moods change. Feelings come and go. In fact, if need be, even try to recall being manic—that in some moments of life, you literally felt on top of the world. The main point to remember is that you will not have to feel depressed forever. That terrible feeling *will* go away.

Once your depression is over, there might be a temptation to belittle yourself. The difference between being depressed and not being depressed can literally seem like night and day, and so you might feel embarrassed or ashamed to have let yourself get so carried away over seemingly so little.

Try not to think this way. Instead, remember that depression is indeed a serious matter. It might have even driven you to the brink of suicide. You should feel proud of yourself for getting the help you needed, when so many other people fail to do so. And the people you care about are proud of you as well, and happy you are still here—even if they do not tell you in so many words.

If you are a creative person, perhaps through writing or painting or music you can convey how you feel now that the depression has subsided. Or you can simply talk about your experiences to those who need to hear them: depressed people, their loved ones, the medical community, and our elected officials who decide what illnesses get funded. Your story might give hope to other people, and also generate public awareness on many levels.

CHAPTER 14

How to Stay in Control

Whether you are bipolar yourself or are close to someone who is, it might feel at times as though your whole life revolves around this serious mood disorder. While bipolar disorder does require considerable attention from both self and loved ones, it does not have to dominate your every thought and action. This chapter contains some ideas for how to keep bipolar disorder from taking over your life, whether you yourself are bipolar or not.

Look at the Bright Side of Bipolar

If you sometimes are overwhelmed by all the do's and don'ts of being bipolar—all the symptoms and medications and possible side effects—it can be helpful to remember positive aspects of all this information. In fact, even treatment can have its benefits, such as increased self-knowledge and incentives to lead a healthy life.

The Positive Aspects of Treatment

If you think of "treatment" simply as pills you have to take every day, and the follow-up visits to a doctor, try thinking of the concept in a broader sense. Whether you are bipolar yourself or are someone close to a bipolar person, there is a wider range of benefits.

First of all, being treated for bipolar involves more knowledge about the self. If you are bipolar, you know quite a lot about what sorts of moods and behaviors are who you "really" are, and what stems from your bipolar disorder. Thus, you are more self-aware than many other people are. And if you also are in therapy, you learn about yourself in those ways as well. A loved one of a bipolar person might also be benefiting from therapy, and can reflect on how she compares and contrasts with a bipolar person—and likewise gain more self-knowledge.

There is also more incentive to lead a healthy life. Watching what you eat, taking healthy supplements, learning relaxation techniques, exercising, getting a good night's sleep, staying away from alcohol and drug abuse . . . the list of things you have been encouraged to do to improve your life as a bipolar person is virtually endless. You can end up knowing quite a lot about nutrition, health, and the human body. A loved one who is accompanying you on the journey can learn all the same things.

Essential

Pursuing treatment introduces you to all sorts of interesting people. Ironically, if bipolar disorder had not been a part of your life, there are worthwhile people you would have missed out on knowing. Whether they are medical professionals, members of a support group, and/or fellow bipolar people, perhaps some of your closest friends will emerge from your experience with the disorder.

Self-discipline is another plus. Before treatment, bipolar people often lead chaotic lives. Treatment means sticking to certain regimes, and it also means that as your mind becomes less cluttered, an orderly life is possible. You might well have been taught strategies for how to accomplish your goals on a given day of life. Perhaps you also are one of the majority of creative people who is more productive for being on medication. Many people—bipolar or not—struggle to have these kinds of skills, and a sense of order in their lives. Once again, these lessons can rub off on the people in your innermost circle.

Aspects Unaffected by Bipolar

Just as you may have gained in some ways from bipolar disorder, there might well be positive or enjoyable things about your life that have nothing to do with bipolar disorder. Make a list of all you are and all you love that would not have changed had you not been bipolar (or had you never known a bipolar person). This list can include personal tastes: Foods, music, movies, colors, and places you love have probably remained unchanged, or have become more vibrant and enjoyable for you since your diagnosis. These things bring you pleasure, regardless of the presence of bipolar disorder in your life.

You also have talents and skills unique to who you are. While it is possible that being bipolar can heighten certain creative expressions, bipolar or not you might well have talents, skills, or abilities that bring fulfillment into your life, and impress other people. Bipolar or not, if you are a wiz at oil painting or tap-dancing or math, it is something to take pride in.

You also have people who care about you, regardless of the fact that you have bipolar disorder. Whether they are family members or friends you have made along the way, these caring relationships can enrich your life and bring it meaning, and that is true for all people, bipolar or not.

Accepting Reality

Bipolar or not, people who fail to come to terms with their own lives are going to have a much rougher time living with themselves, and dealing with other people. No one's life is "perfect," and some wounds heal more easily than others. But it is possible to make peace with the past, and to embrace both the good times and the bad for what they were.

Even people who seem to live charmed, carefree existences are depressed sometimes. Unhappy things happen to everyone. All people suffer disappointment, and everyone has to live with situations or things about themselves that they wish were different. The unhappiness that you have withstood as a bipolar person—or as the loved one of a bipolar person—is part of the fabric of your life. Like anyone else, you have been shaped not only by the moments of pleasure, but by the moments of despair.

It is true that while having manic or depressive episodes you were not in control of your moods, and you therefore said, thought, or did things you might not have chosen to say, think, or do. Still, regardless of why it all happened, it *did* happen. People were sometimes hurt—including yourself—and some have forgiven you and maybe some have not. In the final analysis, the same could be said for anyone.

Likewise, if in loving and caring about a bipolar person you said or did things you now regret—that all really happened, too. You might especially wish you behaved differently before you knew the person was bipolar. Ideally, people do not hurt each other more than they have to, but no one gets through life without hurting other people sometimes.

Painful as mistakes can be, they are a part of you. Over time, you will make more, because you are human. Hopefully, people learn from their mistakes and become kinder souls for having suffered. But no one gets a free ride.

L. Essential

> Some theories of self-identity posit that how you see yourself stems from those you associate with. For example, if you associate mostly with bipolar people and/or their families, then being bipolar is probably the most important part of your identity. If you instead associate mostly with, for example, fellow lawyers, you value being a lawyer more than being bipolar.

Being bipolar—or being close to a bipolar person—can make people have a negative outlook on themselves and the world around them. It is only natural that hardships and disappointments take their toll upon the human spirit. But a negative outlook makes it hard to appreciate good things when they happen.

Mania can make someone feel on the top of the world—but it goes away, and even while it is there it can be dangerous. Even if chronic depression is under control there are everyday disappointments, setbacks, and annoyances that can wound the self. For the bipolar person or his loved ones, there can also be a deep sense of regret about the past, and an apprehension about the future.

In fact, some people become so accustomed to things going wrong that they expect it. And so when a new kind of happiness becomes possible—for example, when a bipolar person responds superbly to treatment—they simply do not know how to accept it. Even if this happiness did not feel so frighteningly unfamiliar, some people might feel guilty and unworthy. They feel they made so many mistakes as a bipolar person—or were so wrong in blaming the bipolar person—that they do not deserve peace, prosperity, and happiness.

It is important to be able to accept the past as part of who you are . . . and then get beyond it. You and your loved ones deserve a fresh start, and a new chance at happiness.

Turn Your Focus to Others

One of the most proven ways of getting out of a rut is to help other people. Even if you already are a caretaker to a bipolar person, there are things you can do for others that will help you have a fresh outlook.

If You Are Bipolar

As a bipolar person, you know a lot about being human—and you might be able to take this understanding and compassionately share it with others. You should not take on anything that might be more than you can handle; it would be wise to check with your doctor first. But even if it is just for a few hours a week, you might be able to do something that not only benefits humankind, but also helps you forget about your own troubles for a little while.

Perhaps you could help others who deal with a topic you are all too familiar with—bipolar disorder. You can become part of a support group or network for bipolar people and their loved ones. Also, you might be able to speak publicly on the topic, to educate others.

But there also are many things you can do that are not directly related to bipolar disorder. You can volunteer to help other kinds of people. For example, perhaps you could read to the blind or the elderly. Or deliver groceries for someone who is infirm. If you do not care to work that directly with people, you could offer to mail envelopes for a social or political cause you feel strongly about. Or you could volunteer to rake leaves in your neighborhood park, or pick up trash at your local beach.

 Fact

Conventional morality means that you do things because you think people will approve of you, or because you value law and order. By contrast, post-conventional morality refers to people who are willing to make real sacrifices for the benefit of humanity. It is much less common than conventional morality, and its rewards are more inner-directed.

If you have time and money to spare, you can organize fundraisers for worthy charities, or simply make donations yourself.

The point is that even if you cannot hold down a job, you might be able to do a little something even just now and then that gives your life more meaning, and makes you feel like a productive citizen.

If You Care for a Bipolar Person

If you already worry about, provide for, or assist a bipolar person, you might be thinking that you already do your fair share of helping other people, thank you very much. If anything, you might need to make more time for yourself.

Nonetheless, you just might find it therapeutic to take your mind off this specific person for a while and worry about or help someone else instead. Doing some form of volunteer work for the disadvantaged, improving your community, or working for a cause you believe in can give you a renewed sense of purpose in life. It can help remind you that there is a world beyond worrying about your loved one.

You still need time just for you. But remember, volunteer work can be a good way to meet interesting new friends. Especially if you have been spending a lot of time focusing on the bipolar person in your life, there might be a lack of people in your life to socialize with. And still another possibility is that you and the bipolar person could volunteer for something *together*.

Learning from Defeat

In striving to get beyond the limitations imposed by bipolar disorder, you may sometimes succeed and other times fail. But beyond success or failure, there is the matter of what you do with it all.

Let's say you have not worked in a while, and then you try a new job. But it is too much for you to handle. A short while later, you either quit or get fired. There are many self-defeating things you can think, including:

- It is all my fault.
- It is all their fault.
- I might as well never even try to work again.
- I am an incompetent person.
- Everyone is always out to get me.
- I will never succeed at anything.

But instead of coming to these hasty, negative conclusions, you can see if there are some specific things for you to learn: What did you do right at the job and what did you have problems with? The things that come easily for you are worth noting. Maybe there is a job out there in which you can do these things only.

Of the things you had trouble with, what if anything can you do to improve your skill? Perhaps some things about the job are simply beyond your level of endurance. But were there other things that with a little more training, or a change in medication, or a slightly different outlook, you might be able to handle in the future? If so, what specific steps can you make to accomplish this?

Did you learn more about a particular type of work? Though your employment was not successful, did you nonetheless learn more about the ins and outs of that particular type of business? Is it possible to apply this information to a future enterprise?

Using the same example of an unsuccessful job experience, are there also larger lessons that you can take away from it? Ask yourself the following questions:

- **Did you learn more about your strengths and weaknesses?** The job notwithstanding, do you now have a deeper awareness of what sorts of environments you can handle, the kinds of situations you find acceptable, and the types of people you find interesting?
- **Did you learn more about how you relate to other people?** Were there people you found it easy to talk to? Difficult to talk to? What made the difference—when are you comfortable in social situations, and when are you uncomfortable?
- **Did you learn more about how to present yourself to others?** In the job interview process, in talking with the boss, or in dealing with co-workers, clients, or the general public, do you now know a little more about what is effective and what is not effective?
- **Did you learn more about how to accept defeat?** No one likes to have something they were looking forward to not work out. But whether you quit or were fired, did this experience teach you anything about how you can be disappointed or hurt, yet still keep trying to have a good life?
- **Did you learn more about how to cheer yourself up?** Since unhappy things happen to everyone, it is no small gift to

know how to how be good to yourself when disappointment strikes.

- **Did you learn more about how to ask others for help?** If you felt embarrassed or ashamed about the job, were you able to get past all that and share with your support network how you really felt? Being able to seek and accept help is another important life skill.
- **Did you learn more about how effective your medication is?** If you have wondered sometimes if your medication does or does not have certain effects on your bipolar disorder, did you learn anything more about this from the job?

Losing a job is just one example. But you can apply this kind of thinking to any number of situations you encounter.

Accepting Limitations

Some bipolar people seem unstoppable. They are famous and successful, and whatever treatment they are on, it certainly would appear to be highly effective. Other bipolar people might be less well known, but are just as successful in their own way.

But then there are other bipolar people who seem to struggle much harder. Treatment is partially effective at best. Even if the medication technically keeps their symptoms away, it might have side effects that make it hard to do other kinds of things. A realistic sense of your limitations can help you to make peace with bipolar disorder—and with your life. The same holds true for the people who care about you—there is only so much you can do, and only so much they can do.

Your Own Limitations

It is always possible that tomorrow will see a new kind of treatment that makes life dramatically easier for the bipolar person. But in the meantime, it can be important to come to terms with what you are able to do, and also what those around you are able to do.

Whether other people think of you as super-human, incompetent, or somewhere in between, as a bipolar person, you might privately wish that you could get past certain kinds of thinking or behavioral patterns. You might wish there were things you were capable of doing that you are not. Perhaps medication seems to impose certain limitations as well.

It is a good idea to remember that everyone has things they wish they were better at, had time for, remembered to do, and so on. Many people wish they could lose twenty pounds, remember to save money for a vacation, or had the nerve to tell off their boss, quit their job, and study painting in Florence. If you have had to compromise some of your life goals or daily habits, you are hardly unique among human-kind. If these compromises had not involved bipolar disorder, other compromises would have been made involving something else.

L., Essential

Having multiple roles in life usually means having multiple social networks. While this can make for a busier daily life, it often reduces stress. By having more than one social network to fall back on, people often worry less if there are problems with one of their networks. Thus, it is often wise to be a diverse person with many interests.

If you are the loved one of a bipolar person, perhaps you are hard on yourself for not figuring out sooner that the person you care about is bipolar. Or maybe you regret having said or done certain things that you feel must have made the person all the more lost and unhappy. You might wish you could do more to help the person—or on the other hand, maybe you worry that you do too much. When you have to deal with the needs of a bipolar person, *plus* the needs of other people at the same time—not to mention your own needs— you might feel as if there is no way to win, no way to please everyone, and you put yourself down for not having some magic solution.

You would be wise to remember that there are no magic answers, and that no one is perfect. The situations you find yourself in would be challenging for anyone. You also might need to remember that your mere words cannot make someone not be bipolar anymore, nor can any sort of strategy you plot.

Others' Limitations

In dealing with bipolar disorder, it also is useful to remember that the *other* people involved have limitations as well.

One of the symptoms of mania is being overly nosy about other people's business. As a bipolar person, it is a good idea to avoid getting obsessed about what the other people in your life are doing "right" or "wrong." By all means speak up if you think someone is (for example) treating you too harshly, or treating you like a baby. But tell the person directly, and keep the focus on yourself—how *you* feel, not what the other person "should" do. Inform the person that though you happen to be bipolar, it does not mean that anyone has to speak to you in such-and-such a way.

If you are the loved one of a bipolar person, it is probably tempting to mentally rearrange the bipolar person's life—to pretend that bipolar disorder has magically vanished from the person's life, whereby from now on she can do any number of things differently. This fantasy shows that you are a caring person; you wish that someone you care about did not have this serious mood disorder. But this way of thinking can keep you from being content with reality. You keep being reminded of an unreal fantasy that makes reality seem inferior. Instead, see if you can focus more on what actually *is*, and finding positive value in it.

At other times, you might wonder if the bipolar person is copping out—if maybe he could accomplish more, or do something differently, but is using being bipolar as an excuse. If so, you should confront him or ask his doctor about it, rather than just letting your resentment fester.

It is also possible that you become so accustomed to noting someone's imperfections that it carries over into your dealings with other people. If you have been accused of being an overly critical person, you might want to give the accusation some serious thought.

 Alert

> The looking-glass self is a concept that refers to the ways in which people judge themselves on the basis of how they think others judge them. If you think that other people are impressed by you, you will be impressed by yourself as well. But if you think others are critical of you, there is a tendency for you to be self-critical.

Just as you are trying your best to deal with life's challenges, so are other people. Give yourself license to make mistakes, but also extend the privilege to other people.

Setting Goals for the Future

In coming to terms with bipolar disorder, it is useful to be forgiving of the past and accepting about the present. But it is also helpful to have realistic goals for the future. These goals can keep you from obsessing or despairing about things not going as you would like today.

For the Bipolar Person

With input from your psychiatrist and psychologist (if you have one), think about what you might be able to improve in your life. A primary thing to examine is your outlook and attitude. If there are negative assumptions you make about yourself, others, or certain situations, is it possible to frame these ideas to make them more productive?

Also consider your job or career. If you do not work at all, is it possible you could find something to do part-time? If you do work, is it something you enjoy, or would you be happier doing something else? If you like what you do, is there a goal you can set for yourself to make your career even more engaging?

In terms of your home environment, ask yourself: Do you have a home that makes you feel good when you enter it? What are some realistic, affordable things you can do to make your home nicer?

In terms of diet and exercise: Do you eat balanced meals? Do you get at least some form of regular exercise, even if it is just walking? Would you like to be in better shape, eat better, or stick to a realistic diet?

 ## Fact

The term "possible selves" refers to how you can mentally imagine yourself taking on different roles from the ones you now occupy. Often, the new roles you choose are ones that you think will be consistent with the self-image you want to have. Roles that dramatically depart from your current self-image might be chosen as a means to reinvent yourself.

Your close personal relationships are another very important part of your life. If you do not have a partner, is it a realistic goal to try to have one? Do you go on dates? If you do have a partner, are there things you can do to improve the relationship? Are there people you would like to get along with better, or apologize to? Are there other people you feel you need to say important things to, or change how you deal with them?

In terms of personal interests: Do you have an interest or hobby that you enjoy? Is there something you would like to spend time doing that you can afford to do, yet you are not doing? Do you ever do volunteer work?

These are just some of the areas you can choose from. By focusing on a realistic future goal, you do not have to dwell quite so much on the ways in which bipolar disorder might confine you. And in the bargain, you might even obtain the goal, and be enriched by it.

For the Loved One of a Bipolar Person

You can think about many of the same issues in setting goals for yourself. Perhaps the main thing to add to the list is how you are treating yourself. Do you tend to think only about the bipolar person in your life, or do you remember to make time (both mental and physical) for your own needs, your own goals and pursuits? If not, then that in itself can become a goal for you: remembering to make time for yourself. Pick something specific to start with, even if it is just that every day you will read a book you enjoy for thirty minutes. Giving yourself this kind of time and space will help you to think of yourself more often.

Taking Social Action

Still another area to consider in improving treatment for bipolar people is social activism. Taking a proactive role for people with mental disorders, and working for more funding and social awareness, can make life easier for bipolar people and their loved ones. Additionally, you might feel a deeper kind of happiness or purpose in life by contributing to worthy causes that are close to your heart. There also are other kinds of social causes that you might have strong feelings about, and which deserve your attention.

Special Volunteering

Other kinds of volunteer work have already been discussed. But there are certain types of needy people that are statistically likely to have a mental disorder. By helping in these areas, you are likely to help other bipolar people.

Homelessness

It is not known exactly how many homeless people there are in the United States. Estimates generally range between a quarter- to a half-million. As previously mentioned, it also is estimated that about a third of these people are homeless because of mental conditions such as bipolar disorder. Unable to work, neglected by family and others, these people lose their address—and with it, the eligibility for government assistance.

Many of these people also have an alcohol or drug addiction. As also discussed earlier, people often turn to drugs or alcohol to lessen the pain of their mental disorder. In some cases, this leads to an inability to function well enough to hold onto a place to live. Still other people might be already homeless because of mental issues, and then develop an alcohol or drug dependency once living on the streets.

Fact

Homelessness in the United States is increasingly a family problem. At present, it is estimated that 36 percent of all homeless situations include children. And this percentage has probably doubled from a decade ago. Higher costs of living would account for some of this increase, along with rises in mental illness and substance abuse.

There are numerous ways you can help homeless people: by making a donation to a bona fide charity that works with the homeless, by volunteering at a homeless shelter, by offering counseling to homeless people (including strategies for getting a residence), and by becoming an advocate for more government funding for homeless people.

Suicide Prevention

The statistics on suicide and mental disorders have already been discussed in Chapter 8. Yet although suicide is one of the major causes of death in the United States, it is seldom discussed alongside heart disease, cancer, and AIDS. Most people who attempt suicide suffer from a mental disorder, yet the misperception persists that suicide is some pure act of individual will. So generally it is not perceived as something potentially "curable," like cancer. However, if these mental disorders were all successfully treated, there would be extremely low rates of suicide attempts. To get to that point, there must be more research—and research, of course, costs money.

There are at least three ways you can take a proactive stance in regard to suicide. One is to start educating your elected officials and the general public on the need for more funding for research on mental disorders. Make these people aware of the social and economic cost of mental illness, and the ways in which suicide could be prevented.

Second, you can similarly share the need for funding for suicide prevention centers and sliding-scale therapy. Or you can make a donation to such a center yourself. (See following section.)

Finally, you can consider offering your time as a suicide prevention counselor. You should first discuss the matter with your own doctor(s), to see if this is a good idea. If given the green light, there probably is a suicide hotline in or near your community that can use volunteers. As a bipolar person (or as someone close to a bipolar person) you might well have a great deal of wisdom to share about how to find meaning in life, how to rebuild your life, and how to regain hope.

Donations and Fundraising

If you have money to spare, you can make a donation to any number of worthy endeavors that help the mentally ill. Or, you can work with a group that raises funds. Either way, you are helping a worthy cause to stay afloat—and that is no small contribution in today's very expensive world.

Making Donations

If you have discretionary funds to spare, you might consider making a donation to local service resources such as a homeless shelter, a suicide prevention center, a mental hospital or halfway house, or a low-cost mental health clinic. You can also give money to mental health organizations and research centers.

Before making a donation, you might want to find out the following:

- How long has this enterprise been in existence?
- Who is it run by, and what are their credentials?
- How much of each dollar donated goes directly to helping people and/or research?

- Is the donation tax deductible?
- Is there a similar organization you could also give money to, and how does it compare with this one?

You might find out some useful information by contacting the National Alliance for the Mentally Ill (*www.nami.org*), or the National Depressive and Manic-Depressive Association (*www.ndmda.org*).

In any case, you should not feel guilty if "all" you can do is give money to a cause you believe in. Without funds, the most worthwhile organization in the world cannot keep going.

Once you give money to one group or cause, it is possible that you will be solicited by organizations that represent similar interests. Groups often pay money for these kinds of computer-generated lists. You should feel free to give or not give to these additional groups as you see fit.

Raising Funds

Charitable and nonprofit organizations offer people numerous ways of raising funds. Besides simple direct solicitation (such as making phone calls), you might be encouraged to hold a fundraiser in your home. You can socialize with friends who make donations to the cause.

Other common strategies include walk-a-thons or bike-a-thons, in which donors pledge a certain number of dollars for each mile you walk or pedal. Still other groups might have donation tables at malls or business districts. Again, these all can be ways of making new friends, besides raising money.

If you are well placed in the business community, you also might consider contacting businesses and corporations to make contributions. Again, this should be done through the direction of the group you are helping.

⌐. Essential

In the United States at present, about $250 billion a year is given to charitable organizations. Of this, about 75 percent comes from private individuals. The rest comes from foundations (12 percent), bequests (8 percent), and corporations (5 percent). So it is mostly individuals who work to make a difference, not giant organizations.

Finally, you can simply share with family and friends the need to make donations—though be careful not to come on too strong. Make them all aware of how and why funding is needed for something, supply them with a way of getting more information, and then leave it at that.

Lobbying for Funding

Elected officials expect to meet with lobbyists—people (often from organized coalitions) who volunteer or are paid to convince the official to vote a particular way on legislation that benefits the lobbyists' cause. The power of lobbyists should not be underestimated. It is often said, for example, that lobbyists for the tobacco industry and the National Rifle Association have a strong impact on public policy regarding the sale of tobacco and gun control.

Becoming a Lobbyist

If you are a persuasive and articulate speaker who can make a good impression, you might consider volunteering sometime to meet with your elected officials on the state or federal level. Before doing so, you should educate yourself as to whether there is any pending legislation that might impact the mentally ill community. Such bills could include proposed cuts or increases in funding for mental health and social work facilities, medical facilities in general, public health assistance, or research on mental illness. You also should educate yourself on the facts surrounding the bill, so that you can intelligently argue why funding mental health issues is a worthwhile use of the taxpayer's dollar. This often means finding out what individuals or groups represent this side of the argument. (If the bill is pro-funding, you can find out who sponsored it.) Such networks often have fact sheets or training sessions to help new lobbyists.

Helping a Lobbyist

If you do not want to be a lobbyist yourself (or if your doctor does not think it a wise idea), you can still support lobbying efforts in several ways. One way is to make a donation to the group or organization that does the lobbying. Another possibility is to offer to do background research on the issue at hand, so that the lobbyists have more information.

 Fact

You can find out what is happening in the U.S. Senate and House of Representatives by going online. Visit *www.senate.gov* and *www.house.gov*. You can look up who your elected officials are, be given e-mail links to contact them, find out what issues and bills are currently being debated on the floor, and also what the schedule is for the current session.

You can also simply write, e-mail, or telephone your legislator(s), to briefly inform them of your support or opposition to a particular bill. Sometimes there are online organizations that handle various causes, and that can even supply you with a prewritten letter to sign. These groups are set up to forward your support to your elected officials.

However, you should avoid signing petitions that are e-mails sent directly to you, and that ask you to add your name to the bottom of the list. There is no way of verifying the signatures, and so these petitions do not have any impact. Sometimes, they are even hoaxes.

Addressing Pharmaceuticals

Treatment for bipolar disorder means medication. And medications are, of course, developed and manufactured by pharmaceutical companies. These companies are a multibillion-dollar industry.

Some Facts about Pharmaceuticals

Prescription drugs account for 10 percent of the health care industry costs per year. Pharmaceuticals are about twice as expensive in the United States as they are in many other affluent nations. It takes the average American three hours of work to earn the money for one prescription refill. The total spending on pharmaceuticals increases by as much as 20 percent a year.

This is not good news for the 15 percent of the people in the United States who have no health insurance. This means that about 42 million people in the United States must pay out-of-pocket for medical treatment. Ethnic minorities are disproportionately represented in these numbers; to be a member of a minority group is to be statistically likely to not have health insurance. However, since most people in the United States are white, most poor (and uninsured) people are also white.

Bipolar people who rely on public assistance receive little incentive to change their situation when it is considered that unless they had a job with health insurance, they would have to pay full cost for their medications. This could run to hundreds of dollars a month.

The pharmaceutical companies themselves often defend high costs as necessary. For example, they maintain that only one in ten thousand experimental drugs eventually gets approved by the Federal Food and Drug Administration (FDA). When the FDA does approve a drug, the process takes an average of twelve to fifteen years. The average FDA-approved drug costs between $500 and $800 million to develop.

In terms of mental illness (such as bipolar disorder), the advancement of pharmaceuticals is necessary in order to eventually have substances available that work for all patients all of the time with a minimum of side effects. Several steps beyond this might be eventually finding a cure, once it is fully and absolutely understood how bipolar disorder works within the brain. But given the high cost of such research, these worthy goals remain out of reach. However, through extremely vigorous lobbying and fundraising this situation might improve.

Advocating Health Insurance and Low-Cost Medications

Other ways to help make prescription drugs more available include advocating for more health insurance. Possibilities here include nationalized health care, or lowered premiums for private health insurance policies through government subsidy.

Still another aspect of pharmaceuticals that is worth addressing is the possibility of offering more low-cost medications. This can happen through more government subsidy for research, and/or more incentives to pharmaceuticals to lower costs.

 Alert

Supporters for socialized medicine argue that most industrialized nations have such a program, and that by not having one, society pays in other ways. Opponents state that the tax base would have to increase enormously to support such a program, and that it also takes away a patient's right to choose a medical professional.

While a relatively small percentage of people are bipolar, the costs of this disorder to society are quite large when one factors in the economic loss to the workplace, or the high risk of suicide and violent crime. If thought of more as a family condition, bipolar disorder can be seen as having a ripple effect that impacts the lives of many non-bipolar people.

The greatest medication ever for treating bipolar disorder will mean nothing if people who need it cannot afford to buy it. Hopeless people who seem "crazy" are unfortunate souls who very much need medication, but have no means of acquiring it.

Education and Public Speaking

Many people understand little about the nature and causes of bipolar disorder, or other mental conditions. They themselves or their loved ones might be afflicted by one of these conditions and not even know it. Moreover, many remain ignorant as to the cost to society imposed every year by mental illness—in terms of dollars, loss of lives, and loss of productivity.

Ways of Educating the Public

Besides efforts such as lobbying and fundraising, you can be an activist by spreading the word—educating the public. This should of course be done in a manner that does *not* suggest a parallel with manic symptoms; you should not be aimlessly shouting on the street by yourself. But advocacy organizations often have outreach and educational campaigns that could give you an opportunity to help raise awareness. Some of these actions do *not* even require you to speak in front of large groups of people. These would include:

- **Display cases in libraries, hospitals, schools, or other public buildings:** Perhaps you can talk to your library, hospital, school, or other public arenas about putting together a display case on a topic such as "What Is Bipolar Disorder?" or "Why Mental Illness Needs More Research Funding."
- **Brochures and pamphlets:** Perhaps there is a group that needs people to compose, design, or distribute literature on the symptoms of different mental conditions, and the resources available for getting help.

- **Information booths:** Large events in parks, town squares, or blocked-off streets often feature information on a variety of public issues. There might be an organization that promotes or advocates mental wellness that can use volunteers to staff such a table. There will probably be brochures available, so if you do not feel confident about speaking on issues, you can simply sit there, smile, and thank the people who stop by.
- **Online:** There are message boards, e-clubs, chat rooms, and blogs available for you to voice your concerns about mental health issues, and the need for more education and funding.

Speaking Out on Issues

If you do want to actually speak out in big way, it again can be productive to do so through a group or organization. For one thing, there is power in numbers, and rather than just representing "yourself," you can instead be presented as part of a larger movement. Also, such groups often provide training for speakers, so you will be able to handle yourself better. The venues can include classrooms, senior centers, town meetings, legislative sessions, and media interviews.

 Fact

Being shy does not have to stop you from making a difference. Some of the famous people in history who are said to have wrestled with shyness throughout their lives include Thomas Jefferson, Abraham Lincoln, Ulysses S. Grant, Theodore Roosevelt, Thomas Edison, Albert Einstein, and Eleanor Roosevelt.

The main point is that you do not have to be world famous to speak out and be heard. For example, your local newspaper or TV station might be interested in you as a human-interest story—as a bipolar person, or as the partner or family member of a bipolar person. The challenges, victories, and defeats that you have known might well be of interest to people, and help to educate them on the realities of bipolar disorder. You can also make a point about how your life is made more challenging because of limited funding for research, the cost of medication, or whatever it is that you are speaking out on.

The same holds true for speaking before government officials. If you are not comfortable dealing with political terminology, leave that to the experts. Instead, talk honestly about your life.

General Activism

The overall quality of life also has an effect on someone's mental well-being. Besides advocating for mental health issues per se, you might want to advocate for other important causes you believe in. Following are just two examples.

Fighting Poverty

With large numbers of bipolar people unable to work, the bipolar community is surely acquainted with poverty. It is difficult for *anyone* to feel good about facing another day of life when they wake up in the morning wondering if they will have enough money to eat until the end of the month—or pay the rent, or keep the heat turned on. And as previously discussed, having a mental condition makes you especially vulnerable to homelessness.

Treating any kind of serious condition costs money. Besides the possible out-of-pocket expense for medication, bipolar people can benefit from a diet and lifestyle that likewise requires them to be at least solvent.

Moreover, as previously discussed, advancing treatment of mental illness can only happen to the extent that funding is available. As long as other matters are given top priority, there will be only so much mental health in this society—which means that many people are destined to remain poor.

If you are poor, or if you are concerned about how easy it can be to become poor, you might feel better if you tried to do something about it.

Whether it is charitable work, community action, or lobbying for different kinds of government programs, you can feel like a more committed and productive citizen. And maybe you can make a difference.

Fighting Prejudice and Discrimination

Also, while bipolar people come from all walks of life, they are well represented by minority groups (as noted in Chapter 4). People are born with a certain proclivity for bipolar tendencies, but often life experience can make these symptoms escalate in intensity. Because of prejudice and discrimination, minority persons are disproportionately likely to live in poverty—and to experience the many strains that go along with it. Thus, it could be argued that prejudice and discrimination contribute to the escalation of bipolar symptoms in many people.

From this point of view, there cannot truly be a world of mental wellness as long as prejudice and discrimination remain. Besides race and ethnicity, people might suffer undo strain on the basis of gender, lifestyle, social class, physical appearance, and disability. Indeed, the mentally ill are among those who are often stigmatized.

 Alert

Some people use the terms, "prejudice" and "discrimination" interchangeably. Accurately, however, "prejudice" is an attitude, and "discrimination" is behavior. Thus, it is possible to be prejudiced against the mentally ill, for example, but if good laws are in place, the prejudiced person might not be able to discriminate against the person in question.

You can help in the ongoing struggle to have a society without prejudice and discrimination. If we had a society in which all people truly were treated equally, at least some of the burden of mental illness would be lifted.

If You Know Someone
Who You Think Is Bipolar

An undiagnosed bipolar person is a serious matter, as she has the potential to cause serious harm to herself or others. It is important to take responsible action if you believe that someone you know is bipolar, but is not getting any help. Otherwise, you or your loved ones could be in serious risk of danger. But your job will not always be easy. And there may be only so much you can do.

Look at Yourself First

Before taking action, it is useful to take a look inside yourself: Why do you think this person is bipolar, and are you truly prepared to deal with it?

Explore Your Motives

Let's say you have a friend or relative who seems to have a serious problem. Sometimes this person can be quite likeable, but then there are other times when he gets angry, arrogant, or withdrawn without any explanation. You get angry and frustrated because the mood shifts seem so unjustified. So it is hard to predict when the changes will happen—which puts you on edge. You find yourself wanting to avoid this person—though this feeling might make you feel guilty. In fact, as angry as this person can make you, you also feel sorry for him. If you ever did try to aggressively confront the person when he gets "that way," you probably regretted it. Nothing seems to help, and all that happens is that you end up feeling angry, hurt, frightened, and sad all at the same time.

To make matters worse, no one else seems willing to do anything about this person. Maybe there is a great deal of denial, and others say that this person has just been working too hard—or maybe they refuse to admit that anything is even the matter. They might even try to put the blame on you: if only you weren't so hard on this person, if only you helped out more around the house, or if only you ate your vegetables, this person would not act out.

It also could be that you and other people *do* talk about how the person seems odd or self-destructive, but it is in a gossipy, negative way. You might even say that the person is "crazy"—but you do it as a put-down, not recognizing the extremely serious implications of what you are saying. But whatever the specifics, this person is not seeking professional help, perhaps never has, and no one is doing anything to try to ensure that the situation changes.

Any number of conditions could make this person so difficult to be around. Maybe it *is* bipolar disorder, but it could also be some other disorder—or maybe some other kind of cognitive, physical, or behavioral problem. But whatever it is, it is important to approach the situation with compassion.

 Fact

In helping others, people often employ the minimax strategy. This means that people try to determine how they can help the most by exerting the least amount of effort. For example, calling 911 when someone is having a serious episode takes just a moment, and will probably be more useful than trying to alter the behavior without knowing what you are doing.

It is absolutely understandable that you would have mixed feelings about this person. You might even feel as though you hate the person sometimes. But it could very well be that what is wrong with the person is something that she cannot control. Even if some—or all—of the problem is purely mental or cognitive, it means there are deeply engrained patterns of thought that are difficult (though not impossible) to change. Despite how the person seems, it could be that she does deeply sense that something is the matter, and might be quite afraid.

It is best not to approach this matter as if trying to punish the person for all the unhappiness she has caused, or to prove that you were "right" all along. You will be much more successful in helping this person if your motive is to *help*.

Prepare for a Struggle

Be ready for a number of challenges if you decide to get involved. First, you might have to do it all alone. It might be that you are the only person who admits this other individual needs to be seen by a doctor and diagnosed. If this is the case, you will need to work hard to stand by your convictions if you want to follow through. Or it also might be that other people agree this person needs help, but you are the only one who is willing to make this happen. If this is the case, you might feel resentment toward the people who could be helping but are choosing not to do so. Either way, a lack of practical or emotional support can make your job harder.

However, you also might have unwanted help. Just as frustrating as having to do it all alone is getting help from someone who is not good at helping. For example, maybe your helper has very poor communication skills, and neither listens well nor speaks well. You might have to carefully weigh whether or not you are better off going it alone.

The person in question will probably resist. If someone has never seen a psychiatrist or in general is highly defensive, he is probably going to resent your interference, and insist that nothing much is the matter. If this person begins bullying or threatening and you back off, that might well be as far as things go.

Additionally, you might be wrong. Since you are not a psychiatrist conducting a formal evaluation, you should be prepared for the possibility that this person will not be diagnosed bipolar—and may well not be diagnosed much of anything else. Perhaps you meant well, but totally misread the situation. This does not mean it was wrong to express concern, however. Even if you were wrong, at least you cared enough to see that the person got help.

Essential

There is evidence that mania sometimes appears in patients with brain tumors, Huntington's disease, multiple sclerosis, and epilepsy. Patients with strokes or serious head injuries might also undergo manic episodes. There is also some evidence that influenza can temporarily create a state of mania.

When to Intervene

In today's world people are quick to label themselves as, for example, coming from a "dysfunctional family"—whereby such statements seem to lose meaning after a while. But if you think someone is bipolar, it is not just a pop psychology game; it is an extremely serious matter. Though you are not a psychiatrist, you still can look for signs that some kind of intervention is needed.

Is the Person Having an Episode?

If someone you know has clearly full-blown manic-depressive episodes, the best time to try to get him help is *right now*. Even if the person is not having an episode at the moment and seems "okay," this may not be true in the near future. It is best to not tempt fate; help the person get help now. If he seems to have more minor episodes of mania or depression, remember that if left untreated these symptoms can develop into Bipolar I.

In today's world, it is often said that people with substance abuse problems must "hit bottom" themselves before they are ready for help. That might be a good philosophy for some problems. But someone in the midst of mania or depression but who does not even *know* that's what is happening is unlikely to recognize what the solution is. Even people who *have* been diagnosed and treated sometimes decide in the moment that nothing is wrong during mania, or that nothing can be fixed during depression. So you can imagine how unlikely it is that someone who has never been diagnosed will seek out treatment on her own. So this is one time in which it is appropriate to mind someone else's business, and get them into treatment. If nothing else, consider it a matter of personal or public safety.

If the person lives with a spouse or relative, involve this third party. But if the bipolar-acting person lives alone, then someone has to intervene before something tragic happens—and it could be that the only person to do so is you.

Is the Person Breaking the Law?

Attempting suicide, assaulting another person, stealing, speeding, creating a public disturbance, and lewd conduct are among the more common ways that someone might break the law during a bipolar episode. (Yes, though some people do not know it, it is illegal to commit or attempt suicide.) The police rightfully should be called when any of these crimes are being committed. Ideally, this will lead to the person finally getting much-needed treatment—and often it does. But it is also possible that the police will not identify the offending behavior as a symptom of bipolar disorder.

 Alert

The often high rate of risky sexual activity among bipolar people makes them more likely to acquire HIV, or experience unwanted pregnancy, than the general population. Other symptoms associated with bipolar disorder can lead to a distorted belief about safe sexual practices.

Thus, if you report to the police someone whom you think is bipolar—or if you know that such a person has been arrested—you should *not* assume that the police will make sure the person is seen by a psychiatrist. Instead, you should inform the police that the person has a history of highly erratic behavior and should be seen by a psychiatrist. You should then follow up, and see if this has happened. You should also report what you know to the person's attorney.

Expressing Your Concerns

If the person has not broken the law, the police can probably still assist in getting an involuntary psychiatric assessment, but they may or may not agree to do so. But you can still try to get this person help. One of the first things you can do in your quest to have a loved one diagnosed is to express your concerns—starting with other people who care about this person.

Share with the Person's Loved Ones

A first step you can take is to discuss the person's situation with his loved ones. If these other people agree with you, perhaps you can form a kind of alliance—to help each other, and to see what you might be able to do to get this person into treatment.

But convincing other people is not always easy. For one thing, you *could* be wrong. But assuming that you have good reason to think that this person is bipolar, it will help your case if you do the following:

- **Make clear that you are not trying to judge anyone.** You are not saying that this person is "bad," or that the loved one did anything wrong. You simply are making an observation as someone who cares.
- **Refer to specific traits of bipolar disorder, and supply examples.** You should make plain the traits of mania and the traits of depression—and the instances in which this person was manic and/or depressed.

- **Pre-empt the expected doubts.** It can be useful if you say in advance, "No, he has not just been working too hard, or feeling happy about being divorced. This is way beyond that, and it's been going on for a long time."
- **Give the other people a chance to share.** Do not totally dominate the conversation. Instead, let the other people offer their own observations. Also, give people a chance to think things over. You might well be telling them more than they can reasonably handle right there on the spot.
- **Have a plan.** If the other people do agree that the person in question might be bipolar—or at least in need of seeing a psychiatrist—they also might think there is nothing they can do about it. It can be helpful if you can say you talked to a doctor or clinic, and supply the advice you were given.

Talk to the Person Directly

You also might decide it is potentially useful to talk to the person directly about what bipolar disorder is, and why you think she should see a doctor. Once again, it is possible that the person will feel insulted, embarrassed, angry, or violated, no matter how carefully you phrase things. Still, if you decide to give it a try, there are a number of issues to consider.

One such issue is whether you would do it alone or with others. If the person in question is a spouse or best friend—or you know for a fact that you have an especially close relationship—perhaps you should talk to her alone. But in other instances, it might be helpful to have one or two others whom the person is also very close to present. On the one hand, you do not want the person to feel ganged up on, but on the other hand you might find it useful to have other people there for more support.

Make sure you know the facts. Once again, you should have a list of symptoms handy, so that the person can see for herself why you are suggesting treatment is needed.

Fact

The boomerang effect refers to what happens when the listener ends up thinking or doing the opposite of what the speaker intended. One of the main causes of the boomerang effect is mistrust of the speaker. Trust is an important thing to remember when trying to explain why you think someone is bipolar—does your audience trust you?

Consider the person's state of mind: Should the person be having an episode, it is extremely doubtful that reasoning with him will prove effective. When the person is in the midst of mania, he will not want to believe anything is the matter—or else might decide you are simply the enemy. If suffering major depression, you might have a hard time getting him to want to talk to you for very long.

Have a concrete and doable plan. Once again, you should not just leave the person hanging. If she agrees to get help, conclude by saying something like: "I'm so glad. Here is the phone number of a good doctor. Let's call him right now." You also could offer to give the person a ride to the doctor.

Formal Interventions

If simply talking to the person's friends or relatives—or to the person himself—is not the appropriate plan of action, you might need to take more formal steps. These can include a group intervention, or legal steps to have the person ordered into treatment by the court.

Group Intervention

A group intervention involves a roomful of loved ones sitting down with a person, and explaining why they feel she desperately needs help. Often, this is done more around issues of addiction or other kinds of compulsive behavior, but it can also be done around mood disorders. The goal of an intervention is for it to end with the person leaving *immediately* for treatment. In the case of a bipolar person, this should mean that they see a doctor that same day, whether in a hospital or in private practice. (This would then involve advanced planning.) If the best that comes from it all is that the person promises to make an appointment to see a psychiatrist, or has an appointment in three weeks, the intervention was not much of a success. Any number of things might happen in the meantime.

Success is never guaranteed. In particular, if someone is having a manic episode they might be *extremely* disinclined to admit they need help, or that anything is wrong. Or, suffering from depression, the person might conclude that he is such an obvious nuisance it is best to end it all. So once again, reasoning is not the best approach if the person is having an episode.

The intervention should be run by a professional facilitator with experience in handling bipolar disorder—not just milder conditions—and who is also knowledgeable about where the person might immediately go for diagnosis and treatment.

Legal Intervention

If it is obvious that someone needs immediate diagnosis and treatment, you might need to take the matter to the courts. This is a last-resort option that is likely to cause extremely volatile emotions. The unwell person might, for example, scream in your face that she hates you and will never forgive you. In fact, you yourself might benefit from therapy or counseling after such an experience. But in the final analysis, it is surely a preferable option to having someone commit suicide—or homicide.

The laws and procedures for so doing can vary across states. They can take hours, days, weeks, or months, depending on the laws where you live, the actions taken by the person in question, and how fast or slow the bureaucracy moves. You can contact your local psychiatric crisis center (if there is one), or speak to an attorney to find the best way to proceed.

Essential

> In some states, it is possible to assign someone's disability payments to a relative or health care professional to help ensure that the person receives treatment for a mental disorder. The person assigned the payment is then obligated to give it to the patient only upon proof of keeping up treatment.

At some point in the process at least one medical doctor must agree that the person in question has a diagnosable illness—bipolar or otherwise—that requires immediate treatment. If the court further concurs, there are numerous possible outcomes, including:

- **Legal guardianship:** You or someone else might be appointed the person's legal guardian. This means that the person is deemed incompetent to make her own decisions, whereby the guardian decides instead. In this way, the guardian can order the person to receive treatment. Should the person refuse to do so, she can be hospitalized at the guardian's request.
- **Outpatient commitment:** The individual in question agrees to follow a treatment regime, and can live at home as long as he continues to do so. Failure to do so means hospitalization.
- **Benevolent coercion:** In this scenario, the person is given a choice between being hospitalized and agreeing to treatment on an outpatient basis. It is similar to outpatient commitment, but it is presented as a matter of choice.
- **Inpatient commitment:** The individual is outright committed to a hospital for treatment. This often transpires when other options have failed.

Dealing with the Aftermath

Whatever the outcome of trying to get someone diagnosed and treated, your work probably has not ended. The dynamic between you and the person in question has changed. Your relationships with fellow loved ones have also probably been altered. For that matter, how you see yourself might also be different now.

Changed Relationship(s)

Perhaps the person you cared about turned out to indeed be diagnosed bipolar, or as having some other serious disorder. Perhaps things never got that far, and the person is still undiagnosed. It is also possible that nothing at all was wrong with the person once he saw a doctor—though hopefully you are not someone who lies or exaggerates about other people.

But these differing outcomes do not necessarily determine how the individual in question or other people (if they got involved) regard you. A hundred doctors can fail to convince certain people that their loved one has a diagnosable mental condition. Such people probably were offended by your efforts to intervene, regardless of the outcome. Some might confront you with their hostility, others might act as if nothing at all happened, while still others might simply lose touch with you.

For different reasons, you are likely to be unhappy with any of these outcomes. People who simply cut you off will hurt your feelings. The denial of people who act like nothing happened will frustrate you. And people who get angry with you are likely to make you angry as well—even if you choose not to confront them.

If any of these people were close friends or relatives before all this happened, it might be wise to let this cool off before deciding anything too definite. Perhaps their feelings will change over time, and you will able to re-forge close ties with them. If these people were more casual acquaintances, you might find it easier to simply move forward without them.

As for the possibly bipolar person: Initial resentment should be expected—even protests of hatred. If the person does require some form of treatment, hopefully over time you will not only be forgiven, but also thanked. However, if the person gets treatment, yet for some reason continues to resent you—again, give the matter time. Let her come around when ready to do so.

If the person never got diagnosed, it might be less likely that even over time your relationship will be repaired. But at the same time, you may want to question why you want to remain in close, active contact with someone you think has a serious mental condition.

How You See Yourself

Whatever the nature of your relationship with another person, part of what you like or do not like about it is who you are in that relationship. When a loved one dies, part of the loss that is grieved is the fact that you will never again be exactly who you were with the deceased.

If someone was close enough to you for you to try to get her medical treatment, it is reasonable to undergo a certain alteration of self. The person may be out of your life altogether, and if still a part of it, the dynamic might well be different. Moreover, your relationships with other people might likewise have ceased, or changed.

Thus, you are not quite who you were before all this happened. It might be useful to join a support group or see a therapist to help you adjust to all these different dynamics. Whether you seem to be everyone's hero or everyone's villain, it is important to keep what other people think of you in perspective.

Protect Yourself

Being in the company of someone you think has a serious mental condition that is not being treated is a highly stressful situation. Efforts—successful or otherwise—to get the person diagnosed are unlikely to go as smoothly as you had hoped. Further adding to the tension is the possibility that it may not be safe for you to continue to be around this person.

Give Yourself Space

You and this other person might be deeply enmeshed. Perhaps you are a couple with children, or lifelong best friends, or business partners. If such is the case, this person and his circle of loved ones will probably continue to be an active part of your life. Should any of these relationships be strained, seek out trusted loved ones, a support group, or a therapist. You need to find ways of not letting this add to your overall stress. Even if you feel closer to certain people for having tried to help this person, you still need to stay on track with your own life and your own goals.

If you have relatively few connections to these people, yet the situation is so stressful that it is causing you to neglect other important areas of your life, you might decide to sever your ties—at least for the time being. You need to make sure you are eating, sleeping, tending to your loved ones, doing your job—whatever it is that is suffering, you need to get it back on track.

Value Your Safety

Once again, it cannot be underemphasized that mania can result in acts of violence toward other people—up to and including homicide. These violent acts can also take the form of vandalism. If you truly believe this person is bipolar, and the person furthermore has never been diagnosed or treated, you need to seriously ask yourself why you persist in this situation. And for as long as you stay in it, you need to make sure you are as protected as possible.

 ## Fact

Of the 2 million people presently incarcerated in the United States, about 20 percent of them have a serious mental illness, and about 40,000 of them are probably bipolar. Thus, while not all mentally ill—or bipolar—people become convicted felons, a disproportionately high percentage of them do.

Always have a charged cell phone on your person when in the company of this possibly bipolar individual. You should program 911 (or a different local emergency number) into the phone for speed dialing.

If the person seems to be having a manic episode in your presence, you should remove yourself from the situation. Should the person turn violent toward you, likewise remove yourself and call 911 immediately. (More about self-protection will be explained in the next chapter.)

If You Know Someone Who Is Bipolar

If someone in your life has been diagnosed with bipolar disorder, the person's ability to stick with treatment—and the success of the treatment—will be crucial factors in your relationship. But there are still other ways in which you will want to concentrate on taking the best possible care of yourself. And it is useful to know when to be realistic and accepting, and when to maintain hope for a change for the better.

Life with a Bipolar Spouse

Being partnered to a bipolar person is seldom dull. It can be a rewarding learning experience, and can have many perfectly pleasant moments as well—but it can also reach a point where you feel that you cannot cope any longer.

Treatment Is Working

If your partner is responding well to treatment—and furthermore does not rebel against staying on medication—then bipolar disorder might seem no different from other treatable medical conditions that a partner might have. Some maintenance is required; at times, choices will be made that help ensure mood stability but are otherwise not preferred. But as couples age, one or both parties often need to take certain medications regularly, or do or not do certain kinds of activities. Medication, doctor's appointments, and so forth, can become a normal part of the couple's routine. There is always a possibility of a future episode—but then, in any relationship there is always a possibility of something going wrong.

In this pleasant scenario, bipolar disorder does not run anybody's life. *All* relationships have their share of problems, but like most relationships the problems here need not center around bipolar disorder. And since bipolar people are often creative, perhaps your relationship is all the more rewarding as you watch your partner excel in his field.

Treatment Is Partially Effective

Life is more complex if your partner has only partial success with medication. You can be grateful for the symptoms that are under control. But if other symptoms are harder to fully control—or if there are side effects that in effect become new symptoms to deal with—your situation will have its share of difficulties. The possibility of a full-scale episode is much more of a reality. On a given day, you reasonably can expect bipolar disorder to be a topic of conversation. Issues such as symptoms, medications, side effects, and doctor visits will be actively present in your mind.

Everyone has idiosyncrasies that annoy other people. But in this situation, it might sometimes be hard to know when the problem is with bipolar disorder, or just the person's personality quirks. For example, if your partner talks too much and interrupts others when they try to interject, is it hypomania (which might not be controllable), or is it simple rudeness (which *is* controllable)? Dialoging with your spouse's doctor will probably help you decide.

Work might also be an issue. Your partner may not be able to work much—or work at all—which will put more of a burden on you. Or maybe your spouse keeps trying to work, but cannot keep a job. Discussions about work and money can afflict all couples, but your situation might be one that will not be resolved—unless you decide it is worth it to part ways.

If you have children, you will probably find yourself sometimes having to do a kind of balancing act between trying to meet your children's needs and trying to help your partner to attain stability of mood. As your children get older, they may start helping you with your spouse, which at times you will appreciate, and at other times you may feel guilty that they are not just having fun like "normal" kids.

Alert

Various side effects to medication, or the possibility of an episode, might place limits on your activities as a couple. Certain pastimes that you enjoy might need to be avoided. There might be times in which you end up not doing something you had looked forward to because of your partner's unexpected manic or depressive episode. You might often feel the need to acquiesce to your spouse to avoid a dramatic mood swing.

In this situation, no one can decide for you if the relationship is worth maintaining. As with any other intimate partnering, you need to weigh the plusses and minuses along with the responsibilities involved. In fairness to your partner, it is not her fault that the right combination of medication has not been found. However, if you have ever felt your safety was seriously threatened by your partner's mood swings, you should give real consideration to parting ways. Even if treatment is only partially effective, there is no guarantee that you will not feel threatened again—and maybe the outcome will be less fortunate next time.

Not Receiving Treatment

If your partner either does not respond to medication, cannot tolerate the side effects, or else is refusing to take it, it is all the more likely that you are not safe living under the same roof as your bipolar spouse. If your partner tried medication but it did not work, it might seem sad or unfair to have to part ways. But unfortunately it might be the only option to ensure your physical safety as well as your own mental well-being. If there are children involved, safety becomes an even bigger issue.

Some people naively believe that with enough "love," their partner will not act out whatever mental disorder she has. It might well be that you can be a positive influence, but in the final analysis you cannot keep bipolar disorder from afflicting your partner.

When mania strikes, your savings might be gone if you do not set up steps to protect it. Rampant sexual activity with partners beside yourself might also occur. Thus, some of the most volatile issues couples can face—money and sex—are likely to occur. And if your partner swings into heavy depression, you might be so fearful of what he might do that you are unable to do or think about anything else.

Essential

> Men with bipolar spouses might need to make more of an effort to develop a support system. In general, women are more likely than men to have a support system outside of the nuclear family unit. Thus, a woman with a bipolar spouse is more likely to already have other people to turn to than a man with a bipolar spouse.

Of course, some people are better in a crisis than others. In fact, some individuals *thrive* on the problems of others, and become quite rigid and controlling as they proceed to "fix" whatever the less stable partner destroyed. Despite their best intentions, such people often inspire strong resentment from others—including their "sick" spouse and their children. Often, if the spouse does get help—if he or she starts taking medication, or a new medication works better—the relationship falls apart. The fixer no longer needs to fix, and so there is nothing to hold the relationship together. Problems are now mutual doings, and the fixer does not like to seem less than perfect.

Thus, whatever else does or does not happen in your relationship with a bipolar person, seek out support groups and counseling for yourself as well. You want to avoid becoming an overly controlling person, and instead have the happy life you deserve. Your children likewise could benefit from having a professional to talk to.

Life with a Bipolar Parent

A child of a bipolar person might sometimes experience role reversal, and feel more like the parent. And once again, success (or failure) with treatment can have a huge impact on how this relationship evolves.

Treatment Is Working

The parent responding successfully to medication can be a perfectly good parent. (Or, if he is *not*, then it could well be for reasons unrelated to being bipolar.) In fact, the suffering that the bipolar person has endured can make for an exceptionally sensitive and wise individual, with a clear sense of what really matters in life. And all of these positive qualities can be applied to parenting. Furthermore, if the bipolar parent has a special talent or skill, he can be a creative mentor for the child.

Children in these situations should still be well educated about what bipolar disorder is. They should be aware of the importance of treatment, and also be taught how to handle certain kinds of emergencies should they ever occur. (A doctor can probably help with this.) But children can have parents with many kinds of special conditions, and if the symptoms are well under control, children (similar to a spouse) can simply adapt to certain routines as needed.

Treatment Is Partially Effective

When the treatment regime is only partially successful, the children will need to be reminded time and again that episodes of disorder are not their fault. Children often feel that if only they did not make their parent angry—or if they could cheer her up more often—none of that frightening or confusing behavior would have happened. In particular, younger children might not understand that there is nothing they can say that will make the parent "snap out of" mania or depression. Counseling and support groups can be especially important for children in these kinds of situations.

Since *some* of the time in *some* ways the parent seems reasonable, the children are able to have at least some good times with him. But this "good news" gets complicated when at other times the parent, for example, belittles the child in an episode of mania or hypomania, or frightens the child by displaying suicidal despair. Obviously, the child needs to learn the difference between what is bipolar disorder and what is the parent's otherwise "normal" range of behavior.

Fact

It is estimated that about 25 percent of all instances of child abuse and neglect in the United States involve mental illness of a parent or primary caregiver. Abusive behavior includes excessive physical, sexual, or emotional punishment; neglect refers to a failure to meet the basic needs of the child in regard to food, shelter, safety, and education.

But at the same time, the child still needs to be respected as a *child*—do not expect too much of her. It is hard enough for adults to fully understand a loved one's bipolar disorder, let alone a six- or eleven-year-old. Adults sometimes feel frustrated, hurt, or angry when dealing with someone's bipolar disorder, so children should certainly have at least as much latitude to express their concerns. Family therapy could prove useful, as it gives each family member the opportunity to be heard.

Not Receiving Treatment

Some people do not know they are bipolar. They might feel extremely guilty about what they put their children through as they struggle to somehow stop having these strange mood swings. Or maybe they do not take medication because it does not work for them, or because of the serious side effects.

But if someone *can* benefit from medication and is choosing not to take it, his competency to parent should be seriously called into question. The courts might need to intervene, to either get the parent on medication—or perhaps find an alternate home environment. If you are aware of a child in such an environment, by all means speak up about it—to other family members, or to a social worker. If need be, children themselves can report this situation.

If the parent cannot take medication or it does not seem to work, hopefully there is a support system in place for the entire family. The bipolar person needs resources, but so do the children. The presence of a second parent can potentially make things easier, but a second parent does not guarantee that the children will be physically or emotionally unharmed. At the very least, such children should have the emotional support of other family members, and professional support as well.

If someone is diagnosed bipolar for the first time after some years of parenting, the children will in many ways be relieved to know what was causing all those episodes. Still, the family needs to get together and communicate. It is a mistake for *any* parent to assume she knows how a child felt about something without actually asking the child— and listening to what he has to say. The family can do this informally, but can also benefit from doing so in a professional setting.

Life with a Bipolar Sibling

Having a bipolar brother or sister can be a source of minor or major tension, depending on various other factors. For example, was the sibling already bipolar when you were growing up? Was it diagnosed and treated, or not? If the bipolar symptoms manifested instead in young adulthood, how much did this impact your own life? Did you live under the same roof at this time? How close are you to this brother or sister? These are just some of the variables to consider.

Treatment Is Working

If your sibling was bipolar as a child, diagnosed and successfully treated, there was of course a fair amount of agony you were spared. Still, there might have been instances before diagnosis that were extremely upsetting for you. Perhaps you felt ignored as your brother or sister acted out such dramatic mood swings and inappropriate behavior. Or maybe you felt guilty for being angry at your sibling, or about all the bad times she endured, once a diagnosis was made.

Even after diagnosis, it is possible to feel guilty that you were for some reason "spared" being bipolar. Or maybe other family members continue to give the bipolar child much more attention. You might have also been expected to help this person a great deal, or even to function almost like a parent toward her. You sometimes might have resented not having more time and space of your own.

 Alert

The causes of sibling abuse in families can include lack of parental supervision or knowledge of children's activities, giving older children inappropriate adult responsibilities, favoring one child over another, not stopping violent behavior, and assuming that the behavior is "normal" sibling rivalry.

If in hindsight your sibling was obviously bipolar growing up, only no one recognized it, you also might feel guilty for not understanding better. Additionally, if your sibling was punished too severely for behavior beyond his control, you might similarly feel extremely sad for him.

In cases where the bipolar symptoms did not emerge until young adulthood, you might have been extremely unprepared to deal with it all. And once again, you might have issues over the attention the sibling gets—or feel guilty that you are not bipolar as well.

The point is that if your brother or sister is responding well to treatment, there should be an opportunity to discuss the wide range of feelings you have toward the situation. It also is a chance to find out more about how your sibling actually feels about these same situations. Both informally and in therapy settings, you can work to gain a better understanding of each other.

Treatment Is Partially Effective

If your brother or sister is able to control some bipolar symptoms but not all, you might find yourself having to help take care of this person. If you are not at all close to the bipolar sibling—or other family members—or if you live some distance away, it might not be an everyday reality.

But if you are close by, you might be expected to at least check in on the bipolar sibling, and perhaps help out as needed, depending on how well he can function. Perhaps you are close to your sibling, and do not mind doing this. On the other hand, you might resent doing it, and wish that you had the nerve to speak up and say so.

There also might be times in which you are simply tired of having to deal with it. You might feel as though you do not have much of a life, because you never know when you might get a call that your brother is hypomanic again, or your sister is dangerously depressed again. Your situation will be exacerbated if you feel that you unfairly are doing more than other close relatives are doing.

Even if you are not very involved in the sibling's everyday life, you might resent the attention he gets—or despair over the way other family members mistreat him. Yet you also might dread an upcoming family event for fear that the sibling will have an episode.

You of course cannot control the fact that the treatment is only partially effective—and your sibling is therefore unable to be as functional as might be desired. What you can do is try to help when you can while remembering to take good care of yourself. It is natural to feel conflicted over such a confusing situation, but you can strive to be clear within yourself as to why you feel the way you do. You owe it to yourself to get the help and answers you need.

Not Receiving Treatment

If your sibling does not receive treatment, there is a strong chance that she will be hospitalized on more than one occasion. Hopefully, she has some strategy for maintaining food and shelter, whether it is family support, public assistance, or her own resources (if one of the rare few who built a successful career before the episodes intensified). But perhaps she is one of the unfortunate many whose mental condition leads to homelessness.

L. Essential

The signs of sibling abuse include one child consistently avoiding contact with another, a child performing abusive behavior during play, an increase in nightmares, changes in sleeping or eating patterns, and inappropriate sexual behavior.

Whether estranged or technically close, you probably do not see your brother or sister very often. This could be a matter of hospitalization, differences in lifestyle choices, or your own volition. When you do get together, you have probably sought to keep a safe distance. Even if technically friendly or interested, one of your eyes is never far from your watch.

If you're in the position of caring for your bipolar sibling as a parent would, then in effect you are no longer siblings but parent and child. You should seriously consider alternate strategies for the care of this person, especially if he simply refuses to take medication.

Life with Bipolar Relatives

Extended relatives such as grandparents, aunts, uncles, and cousins might be people you see frequently or rarely. If any of them are bipolar, they may or may not actively impact your daily life.

Treatment Is Working

In today's world there are people who meet their grandparents, aunts, uncles, or cousins only a few times in their lives. Or even if they do see them somewhat more often, these relatives are not people to whom they feel especially close. So if one of these people is bipolar, but the treatment is effective, you probably seldom even think about it. In fact, it is also possible that you have, for example, a bipolar cousin, but do not know it—if the person's medication is highly effective, and if it was thought there was no reason for you to be told.

But in other families, extended relatives play a more active role. Aunts, uncles, cousins, and grandparents are seen at least once a week—perhaps even on a daily basis. There might be relatively little difference between being cousins and being siblings.

In still other families, divorce, death, or other factors might mean that an aunt, uncle, or grandparent functions like a parent—and a cousin therefore becomes even more like a sibling.

In such scenarios, an extended relative's well-being is more of an issue for you. But as long as the person is responding well to treatment, your burden is probably a relatively light one.

Treatment Is Partially Effective

If an extended relative is bipolar, is only partially helped by treatment, and is someone you are quite close to, you probably have to sort through many of the same issues as if the person were a sibling or parent. For example, if you were raised by an uncle, and your bipolar cousin is like a sister to you, then by all means seek out therapy and support groups. Even if your nuclear family was intact, but you were still very close to this cousin, you still may have your fair share of concerns.

On the other hand, if the bipolar relative in question is someone whom you seldom have occasion to see, you probably are not swept up in the care and well-being of this person. Ideally, you do not wish the person harm, and have some amount of concern for him or her, but it is not a situation that especially touches your life.

Not Receiving Treatment

Once again, if the bipolar person who is not receiving treatment is someone you love like a sibling or parent, you might be quite involved, or at least emotionally invested, in her well-being. You technically might "only" be the person's nephew or granddaughter, yet issues about care or commitment end up involving you. You are just as entitled to therapy and group support as anyone else.

Fact

Family therapy is often recommended in the treatment of a bipolar patient. Young or old, family members meet with a medical professional to learn about bipolar disorder, how it affects their loved one, and how to improve problem-solving skills and communication within the family.

Life with a Bipolar Friend

Friends are people we choose to know. Yet for some people, friends become their real family—they are much closer to these non-relatives than to their blood kin. So a bipolar friend can play just as important a role in your life as a bipolar relative.

Treatment Is Working

Since bipolar disorder is often diagnosed in young adults, perhaps your bipolar friend was already diagnosed and receiving successful treatment by the time you met him. The matter of being bipolar—of needing check-ups and having to take medication—might be something you hear about from time to time. And perhaps the friend has confided about some of the misadventures experienced before receiving treatment. Certainly you are pleased that your friend found the right kind of help, and would be concerned if such ceased to be the case. But there is a good chance that this is as far as it goes. Bipolar disorder has relatively little to do with your life one way or the other.

If you have known your friend since childhood, you no doubt were concerned by some of the behavior you witnessed in the young adult before diagnosis. It must have come as a relief to learn that the behavior had a name, and could be treated. And you also have probably enjoyed having your "old" friend back again.

However, if you met the person during childhood or young adulthood and he was very much having manic and depressive episodes—and you liked the person because he seemed "different" or "exciting"—you might have become *less* interested once treatment began. If such was the case, you may want to look at how and why you go about choosing your friends.

Treatment Is Partially Effective

If your friend's treatment works for some symptoms but not others, you will need to decide how much you can be actively involved with this person and at what cost to yourself. If you genuinely care about the person—if she is like family—and the lingering symptoms do not cause you to compromise what you need to do with your own life, the situation might well be doable. By all means take advantage of support groups or therapy sessions, especially if the friend is someone you see virtually all the time.

⌴ Essential

> Having friends may contribute to longevity. Studies show that people who are socially isolated are 25 to 35 percent more likely to die sooner than people with strong support networks. Especially since more than twice as many people are living single than fifty years ago, friends are a valuable resource.

However, if the friendship is strained because your ability to eat, sleep, work, feel safe, or feel good about yourself is compromised by the bipolar symptoms, you might consider distancing yourself. The bipolar person cannot simply stop these behaviors, and if you are not willing to accept their inevitable presence from time to time, you might need to reconsider your priorities. If this person depends upon you in a major way but you simply cannot handle it anymore, you might feel better if you at least help ensure that there is some other kind of support available to her. Perhaps you contact the person's family, or refer the matter to social services.

Not Receiving Treatment

If you have a friend who is bipolar but not receiving treatment, you should make certain that you do not get involved in any manic-inspired activities that threaten your well-being. If your friend feels insulted or betrayed because you do not want to waste your money, have high-risk sex, go without eating or sleeping, or if he does not even permit you to disagree with him, you can chalk it up to illness and go your own way.

If the friend is deeply depressed, she might well be avoiding you—along with everyone else. You might want to make sure the person is safe if you have not heard from her for a while. But you also need to remember that you cannot "fix" the person, or make the depression vanish.

In the absence of a family member or professional, you might need to take it upon yourself to make sure your friend is hospitalized if and when it becomes necessary for the person's own safety. But the sad truth is that your friend will have needs you cannot reasonably meet. When not having an episode, he might be a very likeable and worthwhile person. But at the very least, you need to be prepared for some rocky times if you become part of his inner circle. And you should also be prepared to sever ties if your personal safety becomes an issue.

Life with a Bipolar Boss or Coworker

If you work side by side with someone known to be bipolar (or at least someone who seems bipolar) the high highs and low lows can take on a special meaning.

Treatment Is Working

If a bipolar person you work with is receiving successful treatment, you might not even know that she is bipolar. If you do know, it might be because you are friends, you need to know for professional reasons, or the bipolar person seeks to educate coworkers.

In any case, whether boss or coworker, the person is probably grateful to have a treatment regime that enables him or her to have a career. This knowledge, combined with the wisdom that comes from having suffered, might well make this person a pleasure to work with. Ideally, she has a job that meshes well with being bipolar: high on creativity and variety, low on repetition.

If there are minor tasks that the person has some problems with, consider that in *any* work situation there are people who do certain things better than others. Likewise, the person might occasionally need a long lunch hour for a doctor's appointment, or need to take a bit of a break. But still again, many people in a work setting might have occasional health needs that must be addressed.

Generally, since the bipolar disorder is well under control, issues you might have with this boss or coworker are likely to be unrelated to bipolar disorder. That he is bipolar might be something to be aware of, in case of an emergency. But you probably will not think about it very often.

Treatment Is Partially Effective

Sometimes a work environment is for one reason or another extremely tolerant of someone's bipolar symptoms. Maybe what the person does at work is not compromised by minor mania or depression, maybe the work setting is sympathetic toward persons with disabilities and makes special accommodations, maybe nepotism is involved, or maybe the work setting is so disorganized (some might say dysfunctional) that the person's erratic behavior seems to blend right in.

But if a coworker is receiving treatment that is only partially effective, there is a definite possibility that he will not be your coworker indefinitely. In many a work situation, there will be a decided lack of sympathy for the unpredictable worker—sometimes out of a general desire to control a worker's performance, and sometimes because the work truly does suffer. Despite what people might know in theory, actually being around someone who for seemingly no good reason is suddenly unable to work properly can compel many a co-worker to complain to the boss. And the boss is likely to be even less sympathetic. Mania can make the person difficult to work with. Depression can mean that the person does not even show up. Ironically, at times mania or hypomania might seem to make the worker seem extremely efficient—and so when it all starts to unravel, the negative impression is all the more pronounced.

 ## Fact

Employers are not allowed to ask job candidates if they have disabilities. If an employer requires a medical examination, it must be given to all applicants. Should a potential employee be shown to have a disability, it must be demonstrated how the disability will prevent him or her from performing the job in order to disqualify the candidate.

Even if the glimpses of bipolar behavior do not cause the person to be fired, she might quit in a moment of manic arrogance or impatience. Similarly, depression can make someone abruptly quit in a desire to get away from everyone and everything.

A boss whose treatment is only partially effective might at times want to work everyone way beyond limits. He might have extremely ambitious plans and goals, and people either get behind them or else think the boss is going too far. Workers might get chastised way beyond what seems appropriate for the slightest lapse in dedication. Or if it is depression that is hard to control, the boss might be "mysteriously" unavailable sometimes. What seemed like a good idea yesterday suddenly is pronounced not worth even trying. *Nothing* seems like a good idea, and it is all anyone can do to convince the boss to not lose hope.

On balance, you might feel that your boss is extremely "interesting" to work for, and if he is highly creative, you might feel it is worth it to tolerate the highs and lows. Otherwise, if it is possible to get a different job, you might feel better about yourself working elsewhere.

Not Receiving Treatment

Unless she owns the business enterprise, a bipolar boss not receiving treatment is likely to be out of a job before too long. Depression can make the person dangerously unavailable, and mania can cause her to make serious mistakes.

If the bipolar boss does own the company (or is the owner's relative), she will probably suffer a high turnover in staff. Many people will find it hard to work for this person for long, given all the inconsistent decisions that are made, and the less attractive aspects of mania. While *any* business is vulnerable to failure, there is an especially good chance that a bipolar business owner will go out of business. There might be bad investments, over-spending, and too many people alienated by the person's manic arrogance and generally erratic behavior.

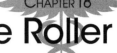

Chapter 18

Riding the Roller Coaster of Someone Else's Moods

You may find yourself the unwitting companion to someone's episode of mania or depression. If so, you will want to keep the bipolar person from harm—but at the same time, also make sure that no harm comes to you. Whether the individual is experiencing mania or depression, this chapter contains some practical steps you can take to protect yourself, the manic individual, and anyone else who might be affected by this unexpected turn of events.

When a Loved One Is Up

If for whatever reason someone you know starts to engage in manic or hypomanic behavior, there are a number of things you can do. Being familiar with the difference between mania and hypomania, as well as Bipolar I versus lesser forms of the disorder, can be extremely helpful.

Minor Situations

Hypomania is, of course, the more minor manifestation of mania. While it can escalate to full- scale mania, by itself it is often not life-threatening. You can be reasonably confident that the situation is under control in the following scenarios:

- **The person generally responds to regular treatment.** If someone is regularly taking medication and regularly seeing a doctor, she still might get slightly overstimulated at times. For example, such people might seem unable to sit still or stop talking. If you ask these people to do a tedious task, they may have trouble concentrating on it. But if that is as serious as it gets, there is probably little cause for alarm.

- **The person is diagnosed as Bipolar II or hyperthymic.** If you have known the person for some time, and the tendency toward driven, highly optimistic, or even grandiose behavior is pretty much the norm—and if for whatever reason you accept this—there is probably no reason to treat the current moment as an exception. (Though of course it is always possible that these symptoms might escalate into something more serious.)

- **Help is on the way.** If you know for an absolute certainty that the person will be seeing his doctor momentarily, you might have little cause for serious worry.

All of that said, it nonetheless may be that you would prefer not to be around the person when she is acting this way. If so, you certainly have every right to make your excuses and depart from the situation.

If you choose to stay in the person's company—or if extricating yourself would be difficult—you can remind yourself that these hypomanic symptoms are beyond the person's control. If you know the person well—and you talk about bipolar disorder—you might just decide to speak up. For example, you could say: "Do you realize you have not stopped talking for fifteen minutes and are not letting me say anything? I think you might need to do something to slow down."

Your words will *not* work like magic, and make it all completely stop. But if the person's manic tendencies are relatively minor, he might be open-minded enough to trust you, and consult a doctor, or do something that in the past has helped to temporarily keep the hypomania under control. It also might be useful to do something together that provides distraction for the person. If nothing else, the person might appreciate the feedback. (However, should the person respond with anger, it could be that the symptoms are escalating toward major mania.)

Major Situations

If for whatever reason the person is engaging in the symptoms associated with full-scale mania, you will want to do what you can to protect all concerned—including yourself.

First of all, you should not do anything that compromises your finances. Even a seemingly innocuous suggestion that the two of you go to lunch could lead to expenditures beyond your means. You should not let the person drive, and you should not rely on her directions to get to an unfamiliar place. If the person engages in even minor illegal behavior, you should at the very least disengage yourself (and you might also consider this an opportunity to get the person help by notifying the police).

 Alert

> If you are sexually intimate with a person exhibiting symptoms of full-scale mania, wait until his moods stabilize before having sex. If you are a platonic friend, decline the invitation to join the person in any misguided, high-risk sexual adventures.

If there is a doctor or other kind of professional whom you can contact to get help, you should do so. You also might want to speak with other family members or loved ones. A serious manic episode can result in extreme misfortune. Even if in the past the person has never caused serious harm to herself or others, there sadly can always be a first time.

A serious manic episode is *not* something you can make go away by being stern with the person, beseeching him to realize what he is doing, or trying to change the subject. It is a serious mental disorder in action, and requires medication—if not hospitalization.

When a Loved One Is Down

Being in the company of a depressed bipolar person is a challenging experience in a different way. Unlike mania, the problem might be how to get the person to care about living.

Minor Situations

If the person is still eating and sleeping, going to work or caring for children (if applicable), engaging in conversations, making decisions, and generally maintaining commitment to the life experience, the depression is less likely to be at the life-threatening level. As with hypomania, you can be fairly confident that the depression will safely pass if the individual is under a doctor's active care.

Nonetheless, relatively minor depression (such as that associated with cyclothymia) is far from a pleasant experience for the bipolar person, or for loved ones. The sense of despondency can permeate the home, as if the person literally walks under a cloud of doom. Others can feel guilty or uncomfortable for not feeling the same way. Efforts to cheer the person do not work, and only make you feel like a failure for trying. There is something very disconfirming in bringing up a topic of interest, and getting an extremely weak, distracted response. You might be made to feel as though you are wounding the person just by talking to him or her. If you are a sensitive person, you might take the cold rejection you feel especially hard.

Hard as it can be in the moment, you need to remember that you did not cause this condition, nor can you make it go away. The unhappiness you feel is a normal response to a chronic disorder. It might be helpful to share your feelings with others who are being exposed to the depression—and to do something nice for yourself.

You can also invite the person out to eat, or to a movie. Outdoor activities can mean fresh air, and sometimes being in nature can give people a larger sense of life. If you want to bring along other people, it might be a good idea to ask the depressed person first if that would be okay. In a state of depression, people are not at their most social. It can be exhausting to have to meet someone new, or make small talk with a casual acquaintance—or someone the depressed person does not like. If the response is something like, "I don't care," it might be best to keep it limited to the two of you.

⌶, Essential

> If the depressed person is someone you truly care about, continue to engage the person in everyday life. Acknowledge that the person feels depressed, and respond with empathy. Do not put yourself in a position of superiority; everyone feels depressed sometimes, and the person might gain more if you shared some of your own moments of pain. But you can still include the person in various activities. If he does not work, perhaps there are errands you need to run, and you would appreciate having some company.

You should *not* expect that any of these pursuits will make the depression go away. But it is useful in many ways to keep the person from totally isolating.

Major Situations

If the situation has advanced to major chronic depression, even a spouse might be more or less off limits. The person might technically be physically present as absolutely needed, but it is evident that he does not feel connected. Otherwise, the person probably tries to limit contact with others as much as possible. Not uncommon is to be off in a bedroom with the door shut, sleeping or staring into space for hours on end. It is actually *painful* to do anything more; it can hurt just to talk to family members about what to have for dinner. If the person has a job, he is always calling in sick, or maybe quits working altogether. People who express concern are brushed aside. They might be told everything is fine, or that the depressed person will be in touch at some later time.

This serious form of depression can lead to a suicide attempt. It is extremely important that this person get professional help. The best thing you can do is to make sure the person gets it.

 Fact

Many communication experts advocate the use of "I messages" when dealing with serious issues with a loved one. Rather than saying that "you" did this or that to "me," people are more likely to be receptive when you keep the emphasis upon yourself, rather than assume you know the other person's intentions.

Beyond this, you can let the person know that you care, that her presence in your life is important and makes a difference. You also can attempt to keep the person actively involved in some sort of everyday pursuit. It is *not* a good idea for the person to be completely isolated.

Taking Action Versus Distancing Yourself

If someone you care about is manic or depressed, you might sometimes feel confused as to when to try to help the person, and when you should instead let the situation be and take care of your own needs. There are no absolute rules, but here are some general suggestions.

When to Speak Up

Though there is nothing you can do to make someone else's mania or depression vanish, in certain scenarios there is certainly nothing to lose by trying to help, and you might even end up helping to save someone's life.

- **The person has stopped taking medication.** There might be certain legal options available to order the person back onto medication, as previously discussed. Otherwise, you at least can make an ultimatum. Depending on the nature of your relationship, you can refuse to live under the same roof, or see each other socially, until the person has resumed treatment.

- **The medical help seems incompetent or inadequate.** If you find out, for example, that the person's regular psychiatrist is out of town for two weeks and did not leave any sort of referral, or you call to say your loved one is suicidal and the doctor does not seem to care, by all means help the person find additional help. If need be, take your loved one to a hospital yourself.

- **The manic person is about to do something dangerous or destructive.** In the throes of arrogant mania, someone might feel indestructible. If you can stop her from doing any number of risky or illegal things, you should feel free to do so. You can also try to get the person to a hospital or to a doctor's office—even if it means deceiving him or her.

- **The depressed person seems on the verge of suicide.** If you cannot take legal steps to get the person into treatment, again do what you have to do to get him to a doctor or to a hospital. You might try by honestly saying that you are taking the person to where help can be provided. But if the suicidal impulse has deeply taken hold, you are likely to be met with powerful resistance—even if on the surface the person acts polite or even smiles.

When to Distance Yourself

Like anyone else, bipolar people appreciate knowing that there are people who care about them. And the help they receive from others can sometimes be what literally saves them. Still, there are situations in which it might be more appropriate to distance yourself—to leave the matter to someone else, or even have the bipolar person resolve it herself.

When the person is responding well to treatment, and has a good network of personal and professional support, you should not feel as though you "have to" stay actively involved in the person's problems.

Everyone has to live their own life, and bipolar people—like anyone else—need to respect other people's right to say, "I'm busy now. Call me next week," or even, "I want to move on, but it was nice to know you."

 Alert

Obviously, you do not want someone you care about to cause serious harm to himself or others. But in an extreme situation, it might be that you cannot help out without putting your own life at risk. For example, if you find out that a bipolar person you know is at home with a loaded gun, yelling and screaming, call the police at once. Do not decide to be a superhero and take it on yourself.

When people need a lot of help and support, it is tempting to try to take over their lives. Sometimes it is hard to know when to stop getting involved. Also, if you are impatient, you might think it easier just to take care of whatever it is by yourself, rather than have the bipolar person possibly mess it all up. In other instances, people simply enjoy bossing other people around.

But if it is something that the bipolar person should work out for herself—or with a spouse or a doctor, and you are neither—let the situation be. Every person has matters that belong only to the self. Give your bipolar loved one the dignity of having an independent identity. If the worst that is happening is that she is making minor mistakes—so does everyone.

Though many bipolar people make good companions, some might be hard for certain other people to take. If you honestly feel as though you cannot help the person anymore, you cannot stand to be interrupted anymore, and that your own sanity and well-being are becoming a concern, then do what you have to do. If you merely pity the bipolar person, your underlying scorn is likely to reveal itself, and you are doing neither yourself nor the bipolar person any favors by pretending to still care.

 Fact

> If you feel endangered by a spouse, ex-spouse, or person you dated, consider filing an Order for Protection (OFP). An OFP will define the restrictions on contact that the other party must obey, as well as the terms of custody and child support, restitution, mandatory counseling, and property and money issues, as applicable. An alternative to an OFP is a Harassment Restraining Order (HRO), which does not require having lived with or dated the harassing party.

Whom Should You Call?

If you sometimes do not know when something is worth bringing to someone else's attention—or whose attention to bring it to—there are certain aspects to examine. For example, it can be useful to put whatever is happening in perspective by knowing about the bipolar person's history of behavior. Keeping an eye out for minor and major changes in the person will also help.

Use the Person's History

Talk to the bipolar person. Even if you are the person's spouse or have known him or her for many years, there may well be a great deal you do *not* know about. For example, let's say the bipolar person is having trouble finishing a task. Rather than assuming you know what this means, ask him or her about it.

Also, talk to other people. This is another obvious point that is all too easy to overlook. Are you *sure* you know all the people that she spends time with? This is not meant to make you into a spy or a gossip. But if, for example, your bipolar person has a close friend whom you barely know, maybe the time has come to change that. You might learn new things about the bipolar person's behavioral patterns.

Additionally, talk to the doctor(s). If you are integral to the person's support system, you probably can be given useful information and insights from the person's doctor or doctors.

If you have a good sense of how the person has dealt with bipolar disorder in the past, it can help you to know what to do in the present and in the future.

Minor Changes

You might want to alert the person's doctor (or social worker) if you notice certain seemingly minor kinds of changes—especially if they are happening more than once. Such issues might include less ability to stay focused; changes in eating, sleeping, or work patterns; changes in sexual behavior; and increased restlessness, agitation, and verbosity. You also might note if the person is veering toward grandiosity, suddenly wants to spend too much money, or is being exceptionally nosy. Depressive symptoms such as listlessness might also be reported.

Use common sense if reporting these minor symptoms. For example, if the bipolar person is suddenly complaining of aches and pains, the smartest thing to do is to encourage him or her to see a medical doctor, to see if there is a physical cause for the pain. Do not automatically assume it is an imagined ache or pain that signals a bipolar episode.

You also might want to share any of these concerns with other people in the bipolar person's inner circle, in order to spread general awareness and also to get input. However, you should not do this in the spirit of gossip or vindictiveness. Stick to the main points, and do not dramatize.

Going off Medication and Other Major Changes

If the person has obviously stopped taking medication, and/or seems to be veering toward a major episode, you absolutely should alert the doctor(s), or other professionals involved. You also should inform other important loved ones. If the person has violated probation or other court-mandated conditions, the proper authorities should be notified for the person's own good. Let the police know if illegal activities are transpiring—also informing them of the person's diagnosis and doctor. If the person has a job, you also might want to inform his employer.

For your own safety and well-being, you might additionally want to notify people in your own support network. If you live with a bipolar person going off medication, you probably should move out, if possible.

Your Protection

If a bipolar person turns violent, there are a number of steps you can take to protect yourself.

If you live with a bipolar person—especially one who has a history of violent behavior—you should safeguard your environment. Even if you do not live together, but the person is a close relative or best friend who stops over frequently, you might want to do the following:

- **Keep drugs and alcohol out of reach.** Except for the bipolar person's medications, and over-the-counter products that you know for a fact do not negatively interact with treatment, keep your own prescription drugs hidden, under lock and key. Do not keep alcoholic beverages in plain view, either.
- **Keep weapons away.** This might sound obvious to some, but a bipolar person prone to violent episodes should not have easy access to a gun. If you feel you must have a gun in the house, keep it hidden, and under lock and key. You also would be wise to keep kitchen and other knives similarly hidden.
- **Have a safe space.** There should be a room in the house that you can hide in if need be, with a strong, effective lock.
- **Do not live under the same roof.** If a loved one assaults you, do not let him or her move back in. If you must see the

person, limit your contacts to public settings, with other people around to serve as witnesses.

If the person is starting to act up in a potentially violent manner, the first thing you should do is call the police. You should have the emergency police number entered into your cell phone for instant, one-touch dialing. If you have police emergency reports in the house, you can fill them out in advance, so that the police can act quickly when they arrive. Include information about the person's diagnosis and doctor.

Essential

Self-defense classes can enable you to have more confidence in your ability to protect yourself. Many argue that women in particular can benefit on many levels from learning how to fend off violent attackers. Your local police department or women's shelter will probably have information on self-defense classes in your area.

Also make an effort to stay out of dangerous spaces. If someone is turning violent, you do not want to be trapped in a kitchen, where there are many opportunities to be injured.

Above all, stay calm: Even if on the inside you are angry or terrified, do not say or do anything to excite the person even more. Say very little; do not repeat yourself if possible, for repetition can be interpreted as your being affected by the bipolar person's threats.

Your Options

If there is a bipolar person in your life, you probably wonder what your options are. You want to help, but you're not sure where the boundaries lie. One of the best things to do is to learn about bipolar disorder. By educating yourself, you can understand what bipolar disorder is and is not, what the symptoms are, and how it is treated. If you can remember this, you can keep from blaming yourself when things do not go as you wished. Similarly, you can also educate other people. In learning about bipolar disorder, and what it means to both you and the person in your life, you can share your knowledge with the people you know, or even in public settings.

You can also learn more about yourself. You can discover more about what your own needs are, and what makes you happy, sad, angry, or fearful. Also, you can learn more about your strengths and weaknesses: what sorts of things are easy for you to say, think, or do, and what things are more challenging.

Ultimately, it is up to the bipolar person to find the best treatment, and to stick to it. It also is up to him to seek therapy, eat and sleep well, stay away from recreational drugs, and do any number of other things to minimize the likelihood of an episode. You cannot control another person; you cannot make him get better or even guarantee that treatment is followed. But what you can do is be a loving and supportive presence. You can have fun together and explore life together, whether as intimate partners, friends, or relatives. Your presence does not determine everything, but it can make a happy difference.

While there are quite a few things you can do for a bipolar person you care about, there are also a number of things you cannot do for a bipolar person.

- **You cannot make the bipolar disorder go away.** This has been stated many times over. You did not cause it, and you cannot cure it.
- **You cannot fully predict if or when an episode will start or end.** You can gain considerable insight into the person's behavioral patterns, but you cannot know for certain what will trigger an episode, or when it will desist.
- **You cannot make an episode go away.** Talking to the person reasonably, or humoring her, will not make the symptoms stop.

- **You cannot make someone having a manic episode calm down.** Mania goes beyond your ability to be a calming influence.
- **You cannot make someone having a depressive episode feel non-depressed.** Likewise, depression will not vanish if you tell a joke, or give the person a pep talk.
- **You cannot control whether or not someone decides to go off of medication.** You can work with professionals and the court system to try to get the person back on medication. But if he simply decided to stop taking it, you obviously were not able to stop it from happening.
- **You cannot guarantee that the bipolar person will never cause harm to herself or others.** Sadly, there is always a possibility that if the person goes off medication, or the medication is not working—or the person simply does not take medication—extreme mania or depression will cause the person to attempt suicide, or assault another person.

It's very important to remember these boundaries for your own safety and peace of mind.

Ongoing Controversies

The treatment of bipolar disorder has come a long way, but it is still a work in progress. More is known about it than ever before, but a great deal remains to be learned. As information unfolds, there are a number of issues that continue to inspire disagreement—be it between research scientists, medical doctors, therapists, or the layperson. Some of these issues might never be settled; whether they are or not, in the meantime they cause considerable controversy.

Bipolar I Versus Other

While it is apparent that various kinds of bipolar disorder involve chemicals and processes within the brain, those who study these phenomena reach differing conclusions as to how these processes should be labeled and classified.

Other Kinds of Bipolar Disorders

At a basic level, there are differences of opinion as to whether Bipolar I is a separate disorder from Bipolar II—not just a more intense variety of the same thing, but actually involving different processes, whereby it should be classified as a separate disease. To use a simple analogy: there are similarities between having a cold and having the flu—and a cold can even *lead to* the flu—yet a cold is *not* the flu. Likewise, some assert that despite the seeming similarities, Bipolar I is a separate disorder from Bipolar II.

Some of this discussion focuses on hypomania. For it is hypomania that largely distinguishes Bipolar I from Bipolar II. You may recall that Bipolar I can involve mania *or* hypomania, and both Bipolar I and Bipolar II involve major depression. But to be diagnosed Bipolar II, there must have been at least one episode of hypomania but never an episode of mania. For mania would signal a diagnosis of Bipolar I.

But what exactly are the causes of this difference? Is it a minor variation in what is essentially the same process, or not? It is known that hypomanic people can develop full-scale mania. But hypomania itself is known to exist at all largely on the basis of self-reports. People who are hypomanic are often not perceived as having a serious problem. When seriously depressed, they often attempt suicide. But such people are unlikely to be rushed to the doctor for being in the midst of hypomania. So what is known to date is limited.

Similarly, there are differences of opinion as to whether or not cyclothymia and/or hyperthymia are truly separate conditions—separate from each other, and separate from Bipolar I or II. And for that matter, questions get raised about people who seem to always have mixed episodes, or people whose only recorded episodes have been mania—are these also yet-to-be-discovered separate conditions?

Still other people argue from a different point of view: that more kinds of symptoms and afflictions need to be *included* within a general classification of bipolar disorder. From this point of view, there are a range of conditions that might emerge from similar processes within the brain. By understanding how they all fit together, new kinds of treatment can emerge.

Indeed, it is the issue of treatment that underlines many of these debates. The more that is specifically known about how all these disorders work, the better the treatment for them can be.

Bipolar Versus Schizophrenia

For a time, virtually all patients who suffered mood extremes or hallucinations were classified schizophrenic. Since the 1970s, there has been a much more distinct category of symptoms under the separate heading of "bipolar," but some doctors and scientists are not yet satisfied with how these distinctions are made when it comes to specificity of diagnosis.

There are a number of similarities between bipolar disorder and schizophrenia. For example, patients diagnosed with either condition can experience hallucinations, and there can be prescribed similar types of antipsychotic prescription drugs. Both illnesses are also associated with genetic components, and have episodes that suggest at least some sensitivity to seasonal changes.

However, there are some interesting differences. Schizophrenia tends to affect men more than bipolar disorder does. And schizophrenic patients are often less able to function outside of hospitalization. This ironically means that bipolar patients can have higher rates of relapse and re-hospitalization. For when a serious episode passes, a bipolar patient is more likely to seem ready for release. Schizophrenics have more problems with neurological functions; they are less associated with creativity than bipolar people are.

 ## Fact

Schizophrenics are somewhat more likely than bipolar patients to have exhibited certain developmental problems growing up, such as poor coordination, learning difficulties, and relatively late motor and language development. But bipolar patients sometimes also exhibit these qualities when young.

Also, when it comes to medications, the bipolar patient appears more fortunate to date. While both kinds of patients respond to antipsychotics, bipolar patients can also respond to mood stabilizers and calcium channel blockers. They also are more likely to respond to ECT. Thus, for bipolar patients, a wider range of symptoms is treatable through a wider range of medical protocols.

Nonetheless, when it comes to hallucinatory stages of illness, the lines between "bipolar" and "schizophrenia" can often seem blurred. A patient heretofore diagnosed purely bipolar might now also be viewed as "schizophrenic," or showing "schizophrenic tendencies." When this happens, is it generally accurate, or is it at least sometimes a misdiagnosis? And how might this multiple diagnosis impact the treatment regime?

Does Stress Really Make a Difference?

There are differing points of view regarding the extent to which things like diet, stress, and home life can actually affect the likelihood of a bipolar episode. While numerous studies show at least some connection, other sources hold to the notion that genetic proclivity and the absence or presence of effective treatment are the sole determining factors.

The Argument Against Stress

One of the issues to consider in regard to bipolar disorder is the difference between a sufficient and a necessary cause for an episode. If something is a necessary cause, it means that a given event cannot transpire without it. On the other hand, a sufficient cause means that it is effective enough to make an event happen, but the event can still happen without it.

For example, when it comes to bipolar disorder, many sources would say that *not* being on medication is *necessary* in order to have a major episode. Maybe the patient has gone off medication, or maybe for one reason or another the patient was never on medication. But either way, if there is a possibility of an episode, one will occur if there is no medication to block or minimize it.

From this same point of view, something like a stressful event could be seen as a sufficient reason for an episode. It can be a contributing factor, but it is not necessary for an episode to occur. Remember that bipolar episodes are *not necessarily* triggered by events. Someone can seem to be having the nicest possible time and for seemingly no reason lapse into mania or depression.

But there are even those who would maintain that a stressful event is more or less irrelevant to a future episode. The argument would be that *every* day has possible stressors, so why would one thing but not another trigger an episode?

The Argument for Stress

Many authorities maintain that stress does indeed contribute to bipolar episodes. Numerous studies have reported high percentages of patients who state that a major stressful event occurred shortly before their last episode.

If some other potentially stressful event did not have the same effect, then it is also true that different things impact different people at different times in different ways. For example, bipolar or not, someone might be devastated that their cat died, yet take in stride that they lost a hundred dollars cash. Yet for the next person, it might be the other way around. The important thing is whether or not the person in question perceives something to be a crisis, not whether everyone else does.

L. Essential

Whatever the relationship of stress to bipolar disorder, some research indicates that the young adults who are often afflicted by it might be college students living away from home for the first time, and trying to adjust to the pressure of fitting in while making good grades. Such persons often experience their first bipolar episode at such a time.

Furthermore, the argument could be made that when it comes to necessary versus sufficient, the point gets muddled in regard to medication. True, without medication there is nothing to prevent an episode—yes, the absence of medication is necessary for some patients to have an episode. But then there are patients for whom medication is only partially effective. These people might still experience some symptoms even though they are taking their medication. And so the issue is quite complicated.

Once again, the debate rages on, not just out of intellectual curiosity, but out of a real concern for how to best treat bipolar disorder.

Anti-Medication/Anti-Psychiatry

It has previously been noted that sometimes people's attitudes toward medication or the psychiatric community become obstacles toward their receiving treatment. But these sentiments also play out in a larger arena of public debate.

Anti-Medication

Some people who have never experienced things like hallucinations or serious mood swings believe that medication is an artificial way of dealing with what is surely nothing more than some psychological issues that need sorting out. If people would simply come to terms with their childhood, or change jobs, or whatever it is that is bothering them, they would not need medication.

Other people are extremely committed to a natural diet and lifestyle. These people believe that there is always a natural remedy for a mental problem, such as vitamins or herbs found in a health food store, combined with diet and exercise.

Either way, these naïve but well-intentioned people do not cause direct harm, unless they refuse medication for themselves or for a loved one who has a serious mental condition. In a broad sense, they perpetuate misunderstanding about mental illness. But they do not try to stop the general momentum toward medication as the answer for mental disorders.

However, other people take things a step farther. They publicly advocate that medication should *never* be used in the treatment of mental disorders. Sometimes, these people speak out as individuals; the Internet, for example, has many a personal web page in which the owner takes a strong anti-medication stance. In other instances, these people are part of a larger, more organized movement.

Some people are extremely mistrustful of the profit motivation of the pharmaceutical industry. In the minds of these people, all the industry cares about is making money, and it will "invent" mental disorders in order to produce a drug to treat them. Thus, these people are highly skeptical when they hear that there is a new kind of medication. They are convinced that it was created only to make money.

 # Fact

Anti-medication sentiments are not limited to the philosophical arena. A number of bills have been introduced on the state and federal levels to limit the usage and availability of prescription drugs, and to make it more difficult for schools and other state agencies to force parents to put their children on medications, or adults to take medication.

It may very well be that the pharmaceutical companies are run as highly competitive businesses that indeed want to maximize profits. But it is also true that it can take decades to get a single new drug approved by the FDA, and that multi-millions of dollars have gone into the research to develop it. Yet whether corporate greed outweighs altruistic motives or not, criticisms launched at pharmaceutical companies can lead some people to conclude that they should not trust—or take—the medication itself.

Religious and other groups that are sometimes labeled "cults" might also have a profoundly anti-medication philosophy. These groups do not merely say that prayer, meditation, reading their books, or attending their seminars can *help* someone who has a serious mental condition. Instead, these groups advocate that no one should take medication, *period*—that *only* the cure prescribed by the group works for anyone *ever*. Often, there is an accompanying ideology that suggests that medication is produced by forces of evil—Satan, extraterrestrials, or other kinds of enemies of the movement.

Anti-Psychiatry

A closely related issue is the general mistrust some people have for psychiatrists. They, too, can be viewed as purely interested in getting rich—and so they prescribe medications that people do not need in order to make them dependent upon the psychiatrist. Many of the same "cult"-like groups that oppose medication also appose psychiatry for many of the same reasons. Psychiatrists—and sometimes psychologists as well—are depicted as purely greedy, or possibly even envoys of Satan, extraterrestrials, and other forces of evil.

Critics of these types of groups offer that psychiatrists and/or psychologists are belittled because they are in direct competition to the group. People join these groups because they feel some kind of lack in their lives, and so they give time and money to the group in order to improve themselves. If instead they give time and money to a psychologist or psychiatrist, the group loses out. So rather than having someone see a professional credentialed and licensed by the social mainstream, these groups instead want people to see their own "professionals" that the groups themselves have trained and empowered to treat others.

 Alert

A controversial aspect of the anti-psychiatry movement is the notion that suicide is a human right. The widespread ethic that suicide is taking a life is said to not apply, since it is one's own life. Others would counter that suicidal feelings do not always last, and that there is not only the loss of the person but loss to loved ones and to society.

Some of these groups attract successful, intelligent people who will swear that the group has helped them. Yet whatever the truth is about these groups, they contribute to the collective mistrust of trained professionals, whereby superstition and misinformation are enabled to persist.

Privacy Issues

When someone is diagnosed bipolar, must the people they closely deal with be told? Should state agencies be told? Should someone have the legal right to keep this information even from a spouse? These are some of the main issues that get raised around privacy and disclosure. Laws can vary considerably in different states, which further complicates the matter.

The Argument for Privacy

There are three main issues that arise in arguing on the side of the patient's right to confidentiality. One is the notion that the state or private individuals might misuse the information. The individual in question might be subjected to prejudice. Others might decide they should stay away from such a person without even knowing him or her. Anytime the bipolar person makes even a minor mistake, people might assume that it is because the person has a serious condition—instead of occasionally being absent-minded or careless, like anyone else.

A known bipolar person might also suffer discrimination. He might be denied employment or housing purely on the basis of being diagnosed bipolar.

The other two main arguments for keeping the information private are somewhat related. The first is the matter of doctor-patient confidentiality. Some professionals feel that it violates the doctor-patient privilege to share the diagnosis with anyone else. So if the patient chooses not to tell anyone, there is nothing more that can or should be done.

Another argument is also about a well-known principle: Many people strongly believe in the right to privacy on all levels. Even if it might be beneficial for relevant others to be informed about the diagnosis, some people would argue that the individual should still have the right not to tell them—and be legally protected from having anyone else do it.

The Argument for Sharing Information

Crimes and other tragedies are often cited in making the case for sharing the information even if the patient does not want to. It is asserted that family members need to be told for their own well-being, as well as for the patient's—and more than simply told, they need to be educated, and get their questions answered. After all, the nature of bipolar disorder is such that patients often do not have a realistic sense of how severe their symptoms are. Informed loved ones can sometimes literally make the difference between life and death.

Moreover, given the genetic nature of bipolar disorder, the argument could be made that the diagnosis does indeed concern close relatives. People have a right to know what sorts of serious conditions run in their families.

 Fact

A proposed new National Health Information Network (NHIN) has the potential to make a patient's full medical history readily available to medical professionals as needed. But this potential asset is being weighed against what some see as a serious threat to a patient's right to privacy.

Also, social workers or medical professionals might benefit from knowing about the patient insofar as tracking the case, monitoring the progress, and so on. The patient can benefit as well. For example, if a social worker knows that an unemployed client is bipolar—as opposed to simply being unemployed—the social worker can address the client's needs more thoroughly.

Additionally, there are workplace situations in which it might be in everyone's best interests to know about the bipolar diagnosis. It can enable the bipolar employee to receive certain accommodations as necessary. And co-workers—or the workplace itself—might benefit from being informed, depending upon the nature of the work.

Forced Treatment

Taking issues of individuality a step further, there is the matter of whether or not someone who is diagnosed bipolar should be forced to receive treatment.

Once again, those who defend the right of someone to not receive treatment for bipolar disorder (or other serious disorders) often argue that a principle is at stake: the right of each individual to make her own decisions regarding the self. Even when there seem to be compelling reasons to force the person into treatment, the question might get raised: Who is next? For maybe tomorrow people will be ordered to take many kinds of medications for many kinds of conditions, given the dangerous precedent set by forcing bipolar people to be medicated.

Adding to this point of view would be the fact that some people do not respond to medication, or else have serious side effects from it. Therefore, perhaps it is not always in the patient's best interest to force treatment.

L. Essential

In January 1999, Andrew Goldstein, a non-medicated schizophrenic, pushed aspiring writer Kendra Webdale into the path of an incoming subway train in New York City. This brutal tragedy led to Kendra's Law in New York State, which enables courts to order outpatients to receive treatment when community safety seems at risk.

In terms of the argument for forced treatment, there are already numerous legal scenarios that enable authorities to make medication a condition of parole or release. Moreover, advocates of forced medication point out that the patient often does not understand how extreme his behavior is. Not only for the good of the patient, but for the safety and well-being of loved ones—and society at large—it might then be part of the greater good to legally insist on treatment. The news abounds with stories of mental patients not on medication who commit serious acts of violence.

The Treatment Advocacy Center (TAC) very much endorses this position, and works to change state laws so that people who are unaware of how serious their mental condition is can be given the benefits of treatment. If you agree with their point of view, you can learn more at: *www.psychlaws.org.*

The Insanity Defense

As anyone who watches TV crime shows knows, the insanity defense argues that a defendant cannot be held accountable for a crime if he was insane at the time of commission—if he did not know right from wrong in that moment. The heinous nature of many violent and sexual crimes causes many people to find this defense repugnant. However, others argue that it is a necessary component of the justice system.

Arguments in Support of the Insanity Defense

It is argued that when someone is truly insane, it is unjust to make the defendant accountable for her actions. It is asserted that it is wrong to punish someone who had no control over doing what she did.

Additionally, in finding the defendant not guilty by reason of insanity, the defendant can then be committed to a psychiatric treatment facility. There, the patient will be safely out of the public's way, and will receive much-needed treatment.

It also could be noted that upward of 16 percent of all state and federal inmates have a serious mental disorder. Thus, the number of mentally ill inmates is disproportionately high, as probably only about

10 percent of the population is seriously mentally ill. Moreover, many people diagnosed bipolar (or with other serious conditions) are incarcerated numerous times over a lifetime. This would indicate one of two things: Either mentally ill people are more likely to be immoral—more likely to do the wrong thing intentionally—or else mentally ill people truly do not always know the difference between right and wrong.

Arguments Against the Insanity Defense

Here, it is argued that even if someone is mentally ill, he can still understand the difference between right and wrong. Obviously, many mentally ill people obey laws and try to be kind to others. So a mere diagnosis of mental illness is not enough to demonstrate a lack of intent.

Also to be considered is the enactment of the crime. Quite often, the meticulous way in which the crime was committed, and the painstaking steps to not get caught, makes it more difficult to convince a jury that the defendant did not know what he was doing.

Furthermore, some people find it unjust to not punish someone for committing a violent act. The target (if still alive), and the target's loved ones are highly unlikely to feel that justice has been served otherwise.

 Fact

For all the controversy it stirs, the insanity defense is used in only about 1 percent of criminal cases, and is successful only about 25 percent of the time. And in about 80 percent of these instances, it is because a plea bargain has been worked out in advance with the prosecution.

Adding to this is a general awareness that confinement to a mental hospital does not always result in long-term success. A patient might be released prematurely, go off medication, or simply be unable to cope in the everyday world. Therefore, some people do not feel comforted or safe knowing that the defendant was instead sent to a mental facility.

All of these controversies will no doubt continue for as long as there is more to be learned about mental illness. And the day in which there is nothing more to learn—if even a possibility—is certainly a long way off.

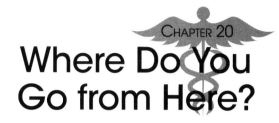

CHAPTER 20

Where Do You Go from Here?

In this book, a great many issues surrounding bipolar disorder have been discussed—including its different forms, its causes, the importance of treatment, and how it affects people's lives. Now, as you prepare for your future, there are a few more ideas to keep in mind. Whether you are bipolar yourself or are close to someone who is, remember all that this diagnosis means—and also the ways in which your life can still be lived happily.

Summing It Up

If you can remember just two things from this entire book, remember that bipolar disorder is an extremely serious diagnosis—and at the same time, remember that it is treatable, and need not rule your life.

Bipolar Disorder Is Serious

To be diagnosed bipolar is to be given one of the most serious mental diagnoses you can be given. If the diagnosis is ignored and your symptoms remain untreated, you could end up in a prison, a mental hospital—or dead by your own hand. You also stand a good chance of being unable to hold down a job, or sustain relationships with other people.

Bipolar disorder goes way beyond the normal shifts of mood experienced by most people. In an episode of mania, you might commit acts of violence against other people, destroy property, lose money, acquire AIDS or other STDs through unsafe sex, and frighten and alienate the people you care about.

If you are not bipolar but are close to someone who is—and this person is not receiving treatment—you might often feel like you are at the mercy of the other person's moods. It might be hard to plan ahead, because you never know when some sort of major mood swing will cause everything to change.

If you are neither bipolar nor know someone who is, you still are affected by it—in terms of your tax dollar, in terms of personal safety, and in terms of loss of productivity to the nation and world. Bipolar disorder is *not* a passing phase in someone's life. It will not go away through wishful thinking, positive thinking, yelling and screaming, or being extra nice. There is no cure, but there is treatment to be had.

Bipolar Disorder Is Treatable

Though there is no cure for bipolar disorder, it is treatable. Medication—usually a combination of medications—can keep the various symptoms under control. These medications can include mood stabilizers, antidepressants, antipsychotics, anti-anxiety drugs, and sleep aids. A large number of patients find a highly effective regime of treatment. For other patients, medication is partially effective. There are also some patients who do not respond to medication, or who cannot take it because of side effects.

 Alert

One of the more recent of many tragedies involving a bipolar person going off medication is the March 2005 story of bipolar patient Tyshan Napoleon. At the age of twenty-seven, after nine months off of his medication, he shot at police officers three times with a sawed-off shotgun before being shot to death by officers.

Medication, to date, is not 100 percent effective. But on balance, it has made an enormous difference in the bipolar community.

Moreover, there is no substitute treatment that has been verified as being nearly as effective. It is a good idea to take vitamins, eat well, exercise, have a nice home, cultivate healthy relationships, and cultivate a philosophy for living. Perhaps most important of all, you might see a psychologist to work on improving your human relations skills. But the bottom line is that none of these things will treat the actual symptoms of bipolar disorder. Only medication will do this—and therapy is also probably essential. Perhaps at some point in the future there will be an alternate treatment just as effective, or even a cure, but at present, medication is as good as it gets.

Staying on medication can be a major challenge for many bipolar people. The nature of the illness is such that people tend to not be aware of how much the mood swings are affecting them. Both mania and depression can seem how you "really" are when they are happening. And after the moods are stabilized for a time, some bipolar people grow tired of having to take medication. Having an episode can start to seem less "bad" than suffering side effects or the sheer monotony of the routine. But again, in part this is because the bipolar person does not always have a full grasp of what she is like when having an episode.

Steer Clear of Excuses

Just in case there still are lingering doubts as to the validity of bipolar disorder as a diagnosable and treatable condition, here are some remaining myths, misconceptions, and excuses that are sometimes offered in an effort to believe that what is going on is anything but bipolar disorder.

Sometimes people try to make it seem that something current in the person's life is being mistaken for bipolar disorder:

- **"Just being dramatic."** You or the other person simply like to overdramatize how good or bad everything is. The afflicted party probably should just take an acting class to get it out of his system.

- **"Just a vivid imagination."** Similarly, you or this other person merely like to make things more intriguing or complex. All that is needed is to take a writing or drawing class in order to express these heightened perceptions.

- **"Just craving attention."** Whether you or someone else, the party in question demands a great deal of attention from other people, and only knows how to get it by acting out. The person simply needs to learn more constructive ways of asking for help, reassurance, or company.

- **"Just been working too hard."** The person in question is extremely easy to anger or upset, has trouble slowing down—or does not move out of bed—because of all the demands of her career.

- **"Just not been working enough."** An old saying is "idle hands are the devil's playthings." Therefore, the problem is that the person has been out of work, or in general does not have enough to do or think about. No wonder he is making such a fuss.

- **"Just upset about other things."** Highly erratic and unpredictable behavior is occurring because of other pressures or problems. Thus, the person is not bipolar but merely recently divorced, involved in a legal dispute, and so on.

In other instances, the excuses given might suggest a more long-term problem, or something out of the past:

- **"Just an unhappy childhood."** The bipolar behavior is not really bipolar but just the kind of acting out that would be expected from someone who suffered serious upheavals during childhood. What is especially tricky here is that past life traumas can in fact exacerbate bipolar symptoms, but it does not mean that there are no bipolar symptoms present.

- **"Just alcohol or drug issues."** Again, this is tricky, as alcohol or drug abuse can also trigger inherent bipolar symptoms. But while it is possible that someone is "only" an alcoholic or drug addict, it is possible to be both an addict and bipolar.

- **"Everyone is this way sometimes."** Everyone has their ups and downs, their good and bad days—and everyone feels a little crazy sometimes. Therefore, there is no reason for alarm.
- **"The person functions, so therefore is okay."** You (or some other person) manage to work, go to school, and/or raise children, so there cannot be a serious mental disorder present. Obviously, all concerned are "just fine."
- **"Just making excuses for yourself."** When people mention that they think they might be bipolar or have been diagnosed as such, others might decide that the person is just looking for an alibi for all of their problematic behavior—an easy way out of taking responsibility for themselves.
- **"Just the latest excuse."** Some people are always reading a book or seeing something on TV about some kind of malady, and deciding they have it. It is possible that these people have other kinds of issues to sort out, but it also is possible that this is a bipolar person searching for an explanation.
- **"Loved ones will worry, or be ashamed."** At the mere thought of possibly being bipolar, some people get extremely concerned over what family and friends will think if they find out. Or maybe someone lectures this person on how important it is that she not "disappoint" loved ones. In either case, an extremely illogical thing can happen: The person decides that since others will disapprove, the bipolar symptoms will simply vanish through willpower.

Bipolar Disorder and the Future

To date, various studies have posited that different chromosomes seem to be involved in the genetic transmission of the proclivity for bipolar disorder. More research is need to hone the collective understanding of precisely which genetic factors are responsible for what, and how these different factors do or do not work in concert. More research is also needed to determine if other genetic factors tend to mitigate the possibility of bipolar disorder.

Furthermore, a great deal has been learned as to the role of neurotransmitters and other processes in causing bipolar episodes to transpire. But as more is learned in the future, treatment can improve.

And while episodes seem to happen over seemingly nothing, some research shows that stress and lifestyle can make a difference, and there also seem to be connections with factors such as seasonal patterns and childbirth.

Essential

Bipolar medications have come a long way. But there is room for improvement. Ideally, there will be medications that treat more symptoms, medications with fewer—if any—side effects, and medications that work for all patients. The possibility of finding a means to actually cause bipolar disorder to no longer exist seems remote at present. But it is a possibility that should not be discounted altogether.

Many millions of dollars have been spent on researching bipolar disorder—genetically, neurologically, in determining the nature of other precipitating factors, and in the development of medications. But many, *many* more millions are needed if any of the goals for the future are to be obtained.

Despite the dismal statistics on suicide, violent crime, cost to the taxpayer, and cost to the economy, bipolar disorder and other serious mental conditions do not seem to attract the same public sympathy as other conditions that afflict fewer people, or might be more preventable. For example, as previously noted, suicide is seldom discussed as a major cause of death, even though it *is*.

Some of this lack of interest can be blamed on ignorance of the facts. Many people do not know the statistics, and moreover they do not understand that serious mental disorders truly cannot be controlled without expensive medical treatment.

Additionally, there is power in numbers, and the seriously mentally ill are a decided minority. The stigma associated with mental disorders—plus of course the nature of the symptoms in many mentally ill patients—gives this community relatively few advocates.

On balance, when government leaders decide how to allocate funds for research, mental illness in general—and bipolar disorder specifically—will be far from the top of the list. Pharmaceutical companies are willing to invest a relatively small percentage of resources on bipolar disorder. But the time and cost involved in developing a new medication make it unlikely that these companies will be earnestly pursuing anything so ambitious as a cure anytime in the future. However, through greater public awareness this situation might start to change.

Finding Role Models

If you are bipolar, still another thing you can do to improve your life is find role models—people who set a good example for you to follow. You do not have to limit it to one person, and moreover, role models can emerge from people in your daily life, or from people you read about.

Bipolar Role Models

There are a number of prominent persons who have been identified as bipolar. If some of these people would appear to be more successful than others in their personal lives, it is also true that some have found much more success after getting diagnosed and treated. In any event, these people demonstrate that it is possible to be bipolar and still achieve your professional goals. Furthermore, some of their life stories are cautionary tales about what can happen to both career and personal life *without* treatment.

But a bipolar person does not have to be famous in order to provide a good example. Perhaps in a support group or network there is a bipolar person who lives the kind of life you would like to have. This does not have to mean that you have the exact same lifestyle or career. But if you look at that person's world and think, "I want that in my own way," then learn what it is that this person does to be such an admirable individual.

This does *not* mean to study the person's every move, or to become a kind of stalker. And it also does not mean that you should get carried away with a manic-like idolatry. But it does mean that you can talk to the person about his life: How does this person deal with various kinds of situations? And if you happen to be around this person when he deals with a situation that you would find extremely difficult, notice how he handles it. For example, if this person seems to manage anger in a more balanced way than you do, what is different?

Non-Bipolar Role Models

Obviously, no one is just one thing—and a bipolar person is more than just bipolar. So there is no reason why you could not also turn to non-bipolar people for role models. Once again, these role models can emerge from your immediate circle, or be famous people that you read about.

If you have a career, or even aspire toward one, perhaps there are people in your field that you would like to emulate in your own way. You should be realistic; do not try to emulate anyone that it is impossible for you to emulate. But even when someone seems immeasurably successful next to you, you might be able to apply something about his or her life to your own, on your own scale.

 Alert

A woman named Mary Karch was diagnosed bipolar, but stopped taking her medication because of the side effects. In March 1999, she murdered her infant daughter, and then attempted to murder her young son. Hers is another tragic example of what can happen to a seemingly good person who stops taking medication.

As for your personal life, there again might be people you either know or read about who have the kind of happiness you want. If you know these people, try to find out directly how they do it. A happy home life does not simply appear; it takes effort. What sorts of communication skills or attitudes do these people have that you can learn from? If the people you admire here are celebrities, you can at least read about them, and see what they have to say.

You Are Never Alone

It is not uncommon for people to think that they are the only person who has ever felt a certain way. But this can especially be the case when it comes to mental disorders. Because there is still so much shame and discomfort surrounding these issues, people often keep their innermost fears about the illness to themselves. But increasingly there is an environment that enables people to be more open about who they are.

For Bipolar People

Besides the several million people with bipolar disorder, there are any number of other disorders and mental conditions that signal the opportunity to network with kindred spirits. There are also millions of people who have never been diagnosed with anything serious, but who are no strangers to depression and stress.

In Appendix B you will find a list of organizations you can contact for support, information, and opportunities to network with fellow travelers. You might also contact your local public library or hospital, or ask your doctor about groups you can join.

The main point is that whatever you are going through, and wherever you have been, there *are* people who know in their own way what it is like. Finding people who understand you in a very deep way can make an enormous difference in how you feel about your life.

For the Loved Ones of Bipolar People

Likewise, there is a growing understanding that bipolar disorder should be treated as a family condition. You should consider it your right and responsibility to get all the information—and therapy—that you need in order to have a happy home life and feel good about yourself. There is probably a way that you can engage all relevant family members in a therapeutic climate with a psychologist or psychiatrist.

 Fact

> Lizzie Simon was an honor student about to go to Columbia University at seventeen. She had her first major bipolar episode studying abroad in Paris. But she responded immediately to lithium treatment, and has since written *Detour,* a popular book about being bipolar that led to an MTV special entitled, *True Life: I'm Bipolar.*

You also should consider networking with other people who have bipolar family members. Through support groups, or even Internet chat rooms, you can find out useful information and receive a great deal of empathy from people who know what you are going through in their own way.

Symptoms Checklists

Use the following checklists for reference as you increase your understanding of the symptoms associated with different kinds of bipolar disorders. Note the symptoms you may be suffering from and be sure to explain them to your doctor.

Manic Episodes

- ❏ Rapid, possibly incomprehensible speech; hoarseness
- ❏ Euphoria that rapidly changes to hostility or anger
- ❏ Grandiose vision of self
- ❏ Delusions of persecution
- ❏ Denial, poor judgment, lack of introspection
- ❏ Limitless energy
- ❏ Sleep very little yet not tired
- ❏ Heightened perceptions
- ❏ Easily distracted; extremely short attention span
- ❏ Risk-taking, wasting money
- ❏ Exceptionally strong sex drive
- ❏ Intense lack of inhibition
- ❏ Thoughts either sharp or dull, changing for no reason

Depressive Episodes

- ❏ Wanting to stay in bed for one or more days without being physically ill
- ❏ Sleeping more than normal, or exhausted yet unable to sleep
- ❏ Aches and pains with no apparent physical origin
- ❏ Major changes in appetite
- ❏ Lethargic, low energy
- ❏ Lack of interest or pleasure in usual pursuits
- ❏ Avoiding daily responsibilities
- ❏ Social withdrawal
- ❏ Feelings of guilt and worthlessness
- ❏ Difficulty making decisions
- ❏ Hostile, quick to anger
- ❏ Deep, constant sadness
- ❏ Sudden outburst (such as crying) for seemingly no reason
- ❏ Pessimism, hopelessness, and anxiety
- ❏ Suicidal thoughts or attempt

Hypomanic Episodes

- ❏ Unusually high confidence
- ❏ Less need for sleep
- ❏ More talkative than usual
- ❏ Thoughts faster than usual
- ❏ More easily distracted than usual
- ❏ More concerned with goals than usual
- ❏ More inclined to take risks than usual
- ❏ More interested in sex than usual
- ❏ You feel what you say and do is not usual for you
- ❏ Other people say you are not being your usual self, or not acting normally

Mixed Episodes

❏ Extremely rapid shifts between mania and depression

Mixed Mania

❏ Episodes consist of a blend of mania (or hypomania) and depression

Cyclothymia

❏ Moods only high or low, changing for no reason
❏ Energy level only high or low, changing for no reason
❏ Thoughts either sharp or dull, changing for no reason
❏ Perceptions either vivid or limp, changing for no reason
❏ Strong emotions
❏ Urges to take risks or stand out
❏ Difficulty finishing things

Hyperthymia:

Long-term, non-episodic presence of at least several of the following traits:

❏ Energetic, optimistic, exuberant
❏ Confident and self-reliant
❏ Always ready for action and novelty
❏ Wide range of interests
❏ Always making plans
❏ Never needs much sleep
❏ High sex drive
❏ Lacking inhibitions
❏ Overly concerned with others

Additional Resources

Organizations and Support Groups

Bipolar Significant Others
For the partners of bipolar people.
www.bpso.org

Bipolar World
A good source for information and support.
www.bipolarworld.net

Depression and Bipolar Support Alliance
A leading national group.
www.dbsalliance.org

Depression-Guide.Com
A good resource for depression information.
www.depression-guide.com

Friendshipnetwork.org
A good online meeting place for bipolar people.
www.friendshipnetwork.org

Healthy Place Bipolar Community
A good online meeting place for bipolar people.
www.healthyplace.com

Hypomanic.com
Specializing in hypomania.
www.hypomanic.com

Mixed Nuts
A good online meeting place for bipolar people.
www.mixednuts.net

National Alliance for the Mentally Ill
A leading advocacy group.
www.nami.org

National Depressive and Manic-Depressive Association
Another strong national alliance.
www.ndmda.org

Pendulum Resources
A good information source.
www.pendulum.org

Books

Behrman, Andy. *Electroboy: A Memoir of Mania* (New York: Random House Trade Paperbacks, 2003).

Conner, Avery Z. *Fevers of the Mind* (Frederick, MD: PublishAmerica, 2002).

Duke, Patty. *Brilliant Madness: Living with Manic Depressive Illness* (New York: Bantam, 1993).

———. *Call Me Anna: The Autobiography of Patty Duke* (New York: Bantam, 1988).

Hinshaw, Stephen P. *The Years of Silence Are Past: My Father's Life with Bipolar Disorder* (Cambridge: Cambridge University Press, 2002).

Jamison, Kay Redfield. *Touched with Fire: Manic Depressive Illness and the Artistic Temperament* (New York: Free Press, 1996).

————. *An Unquiet Mind: A Memoir of Moods and Madness* (New York: Vintage, 1997).

Shannon, Fay Joy. *Manic by Midnight* (Frederick, MD: PublishAmerica, 2000).

Simon, Lizzie. *Detour: My Bipolar Road Trip in 4-D* (New York: Washington Square Press, 2003).

Pollard, Mark. *In Small Doses: A Memoir about Accepting and Living with Bipolar Disorder* (Mill Valley, CA: Vision Books International, 2004).

Index

A

Abuse, 63–64

Acceptance, of diagnosis, 89–90, 121, 197–99

Aches, imaginary, 20

Activism. *See* Social action

AD/HD (attention deficit hyperactivity disorder), 33–36, 53

Age, 44–45

Alcohol, 110–11, 196, 209–10

Analytic psychotherapy, 91–92

Anger, inappropriate, 19, 39–40

Anhedonia, 15

Anti-anxiety drugs, 83–84

Antidepressants, 76–80
  bupropion hydrochloride (Wellbutrin), 79
  duloxetine (Cymbalta), 80
  MAOIs, 77–78
  mirtazapine (Remeron), 79–80
  nephazodone (Serzone), 79–80
  newer, 79–80
  SSRIs, 76–77
  stimulants, 78
  tricyclic (TCAs), 78
  venlafaxine (Effexor), 79

Anti-medication sentiments, 272–73

Anti-psychiatry sentiments, 274–75

Antipsychotics, 80–83

Arrogance, 19. *See also* Grandiosity

Attention deficit hyperactivity disorder (AD/HD), 33–36, 53

B

Behavior
  extremes, 21
  sudden changes, 19

Behavioral therapy, 92

Benzodiazepines, 85–86

Bipolar disorder
  acceptance of, 89–90, 121, 197–99
  additional disorders with, 115–16
  bright side of, 195–97
  defined, x–xi, 1–2
  evolving knowledge of, 26–28
  excuses/myths, 283–85
  future and, 285–87
  history of, 1–2, 52
  mood disorders compared to. *See* Mood disorders
  in perspective, 54–55
  research, 285–87
  seriousness of, 281–82
  things not affected by, 197
  treatability of, 282–83. *See also* Treatment
  trends, 27
  undiagnosed cases. *See* Confronting undiagnosed individuals
  variations, 9–15

Bipolar I vs. Bipolar II, 3–4, 28, 267–68

Bipolar III, 4

Books, 295–96

Borderline Personality Disorder (BPD), 30–33, 75

Bosses (bipolar), working with, 248–51

The Everything® Health Guide Series

Supportive advice. Real answers.

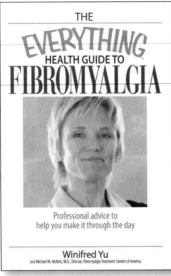

THE

EVERYTHING
HEALTH GUIDE TO
FIBROMYALGIA

Professional advice to
help you make it through the day

Winifred Yu
and Michael M. McNett, M.D., Director, Fibromyalgia Treatment Centers of America

Trade Paperback
ISBN: 1-59337-586-7
$14.95 ($19.95 CAN)

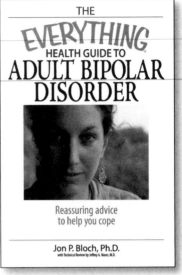

THE

EVERYTHING
HEALTH GUIDE TO
ADULT BIPOLAR
DISORDER

Reassuring advice
to help you cope

Jon P. Bloch, Ph.D.
with Technical Review by Jeffrey A. Naser, M.D.

Trade Paperback
ISBN: 1-59337-585-9
$14.95 ($19.95 CAN)

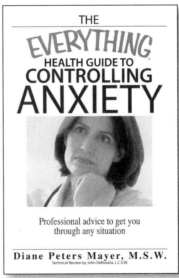

THE

EVERYTHING
HEALTH GUIDE TO
CONTROLLING
ANXIETY

Professional advice to get you
through any situation

Diane Peters Mayer, M.S.W.
Technical Review by John DeRosalia, L.C.S.W.

Trade Paperback
ISBN: 1-59337-429-1
$14.95 ($19.95 CAN)